THE ORTHODONTIC ROADMAP

GUIDELINES FOR THE DIAGNOSIS AND TREATMENT OF ORTHODONTIC MALOCCLUSIONS

Prof. Dr. Ahmad M.A. Ismail

To order additional copies of this book, contact
Toll Free +65 3165 7531 (Singapore)
Toll Free +60 3 3099 4412 (Malaysia)
www.partridgepublishing.com/singapore
orders.singapore@partridgepublishing.com

ISBN
978-1-5437-7476-4 (sc)
978-1-5437-7475-7 (hc)
978-1-5437-7474-0 (e)

Print information available on the last page.

08/22/2023

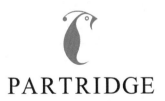

PARTRIDGE

THE ORTHODONTIC ROADMAP

GUIDELINES FOR THE DIAGNOSIS AND TREATMENT OF ORTHODONTIC MALOCCLUSIONS

Prof.Dr. Ahmad M.A. Ismail

CONTENTS

ACKNOWLEDGEMENT/ CONTRIBUTORS

I am extremely grateful to all my colleagues and residents in the department of orthodontics for their help and motivation to make this book possible.

I would like to particularly thank my resident orthodontist.

Batch of 2021 (fall)

Raghda El-Zoheiry, Amna Ali, Yara Abazaid and Fuoad Kawaf

Batch of 2022 (fall)

Dina Alkindi, Racha Alniazi, Eman Alabdouli, Alyaa Alhmoudi

Batch of 2023 (spring)

Jensyll Rodrigues, Maei Al Ali, Reem Al Hashmi, Mariam Alsamman, Omar Alaskari, Sondos Awad

Batch of 2023 (fall)

Ioannis Anagnostopoulos, Emmanouil Evangelopoulos, Ghazwan Al-falahi, Sharon George, Sina Kazemmousavi

PREFACE

This book has been primarily written for the benefit of the postgraduate orthodontic student but may well be an appropriate refresher for the orthodontic specialist. This book aims to help guide the clinician to the correct diagnosis & treatment plan for every malocclusion that an orthodontist may be faced with.

INTRODUCTION

Every orthodontist requires a guideline in order to establish a correct diagnosis, and thereby allowing for the development of the most effective and efficient treatment. Due to the rapid development of dental and orthodontic technology over the last few decades, there are a multitude of new and old techniques that could be used for the various malocclusions. For this reason, proper diagnosis is essential in order to make the correct treatment choices, not only in terms of appliances, but even more so for the ideal timing of treatment. Treating patients using the correct appliance at the correct time will lead to effective and efficient treatment and will aid in the next important phase- retention. Depending on the specific case, the malocclusion, and the age of the patient, we may decide to stage the treatment in phases, thus taking advantage of the vital factor of growth which can influence the treatment outcome. For the above reasons, using our humble 40 years of experience, we will attempt to classify the treatment according to age and malocclusion and discuss the best ways to deal with each as far as the treatment modalities are concerned.

This chart serves as a reminder about the growth pattern in for Boys & Girls (figure 1 and 2)

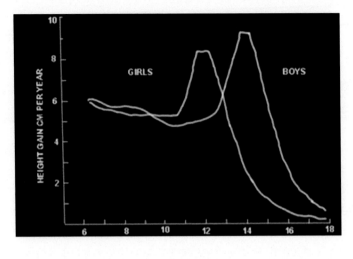

Fig.1

The growth chart allows us to decide the exact age for the correct treatment and appliances used to deal with the malocclusion of each patient, whether male or female. (Phase one, Phase two or Phase three)

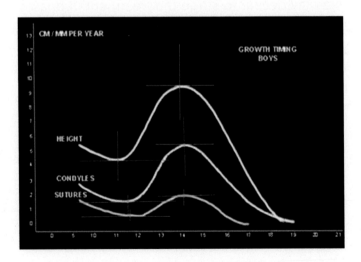

Fig. 2

This chart shows that the height, condyles and sutures have the same peak growth.

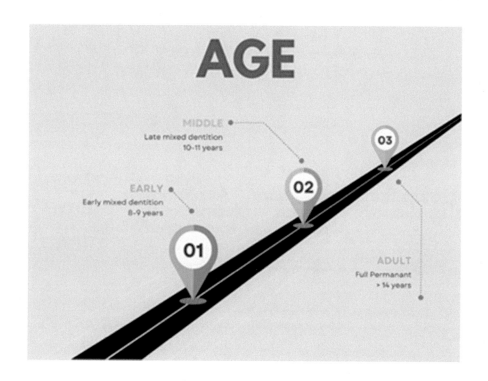

TREATMENT

Removable appliance • Myofunction al appliance • Clear aligner	E.O.T (head gears & face mask)	Fixed Appliance (upper arch, lower arch)	Anchorage • TADs • TPA

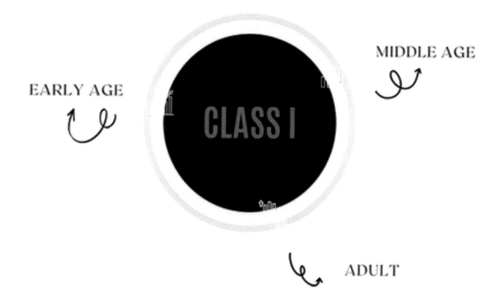

EARLY AGE

MIDDLE AGE

CLASS I

ADULT

Class I malocclusion is the most common type of malocclusion observed in most population groups. Angle's class I malocclusion is a condition in which malalignment of teeth is present with a class I molar relationship (mesiobuccal cusp of permanent maxillary first molar occludes in the mesiobuccal developmental groove of mandibular first permanent molar). Angle's class I malocclusion may present with a variety of tooth malpositions such as crowding, spacing, rotations, bimaxillary protrusion, bimaxillary retrusion, crossbite and open bite. Management of class I malocclusion is aimed at correcting the malocclusion present, while maintaining the existing class I molar relationship which is considered to be the normal molar relationship. The diagnosis, treatment planning and selection of appliances used in the treatment and retention of these problems are discussed in this chapter.

MANAGEMENT OF CLASS I MALOCCLUSION WITH CROWDING

Crowding is by far the most common complaint for which patients seeks orthodontic treatment, especially that of the anterior region which compromises facial aesthetics. Crowding may be associated with class I, class II and class III malocclusion. Management of crowding in class I malocclusion is described in this chapter.

Arch length—Tooth material discrepancy where, tooth material is more than the arch length can lead to crowding. Crowding may be seen in anterior or posterior regions of one or both the dental arches. It may be mild or severe, unilateral or bilateral, localized or generalized.

Etiological Factors

Crowding may be caused due to a number of causes.

Multiple factors act together in many cases.

- Arch length—Tooth material discrepancy, where arch length is lesser than tooth material that leads to the crowding of teeth.
- Premature loss of deciduous teeth.
- Prolonged retention of deciduous teeth.
- Presence of supernumerary teeth.
- Macrodontic teeth.
- Altered path of eruption.
- Delayed eruption of permanent teeth.
- Trauma.
- Gemination of teeth.

Clinical Features

- Crowding may be present unilaterally or bilaterally in the dental arches.
- Crowding may be localized or generalized.
- There is often difficulty in maintenance of good oral hygiene due to inaccessibility of certain tooth surfaces in crowded areas to toothbrush.
- Food impaction may occur.
- Halitosis may be present.
- Gingivitis and periodontitis may occur.

Diagnosis

- Clinical examination reveals the extent and location of crowding.
- Model analysis is needed for determining the arch length and tooth material discrepancy.
- Radiographic examination helps in evaluating any trauma, bony pathology and unerupted teeth.

Treatment

Relief of Crowding by Gaining Space

Space is required for the relief of crowding in the arch.

The required amount of space may be gained by proximal stripping, arch expansion (e.g. Quad helix appliance), distalization of molars and proclination of anteriors or extraction of teeth.

I. Treatment using removable orthodontic appliance:

The following removable orthodontic appliances are used to relieve crowding in the arches:

a. Removable orthodontic appliances with Jack screw.

b. Removable orthodontic appliances with canine retractor.

c. Removable orthodontic appliances with "Z" spring.

d. Removable orthodontic appliances with Jack screw: Removable orthodontic appliance incorporates.

   a) Jack screw in the midpalatal raphe region. On activation of screw, there will be opening up of mid-palatal suture and spacing in the midline between centrals, later this space can be utilized to relieve crowding in the dental arches.

b) Removable orthodontic appliances with canine retractor: Removable orthodontic appliance with canine retractors can be used in selected cases.

c) Activation of canine retractor brings about distal movement of canine leaving behind space distal to lateral incisor and mesial to canine, this space later can be used to relieve crowding in the dental arches.

d) Removable orthodontic appliances with "Z" spring:

e) Crowding in the anterior segments caused due to palatally erupted lateral incisor can be managed with removable orthodontic appliance with "Z" springs. "Z" spring fabricated on lateral incisor, on activation brings about labial movement of lateral incisor to the final alignment on the dental arches.

II.   Treatment using fixed orthodontic appliance:

Fixed Orthodontic appliance with NiTi arch wire or open coil spring can be used to relieve crowding in the arch.

Therapeutic extraction of certain teeth may be needed to gain the required space.

MANAGEMENT OF CLASS I MALOCCLUSION WITH SPACING

Arch length—Tooth material discrepancy where, tooth material is less than arch length can lead to spacing.

Spacing may be seen in one or both dental arches. Spacing may be localized or generalized, unilateral or bilateral in the dental arches. Spacing present between the two permanent maxillary centrals in the midline is referred as midline diastema.

Spacing may be caused by oral habits such as thumb sucking/digit sucking and tongue thrusting. Other causes of spacing include large tongue, relative microdontia and macrognathia. Correction of spacing involves identification and removal of etiological factors followed by consolidation of space using removable or fixed orthodontic appliance or by conservative approach.

Etiological Factors

1. Arch length—Tooth material discrepancy, where arch length is more than the tooth material can lead to Spacing.

2. Oral habits:
   - Thumb sucking.
   - Tongue thrusting.

3. Abnormal tooth form:
   - Peg-shaped maxillary permanent lateral incisors

4. Abnormally large tongue exerting pressure on teeth may cause spacing:
   - Macroglossia

5. Abnormal tooth size:
   - Microdontia

6. Anomalies in number of teeth:
   - Oligodontia
   - Partial anodontia

7. Bony pathologies like cystic lesions, odontomes.

8. Congenitally missing teeth

9. Premature loss of permanent teeth.

10. Soft tissue abnormalities:
    - Abnormal labial frenum attachment

11. Prolonged retention of deciduous teeth.

Clinical Features of Class I Malocclusion with Spacing

- Spacing may be present in one or both the dental arches.
- Spacing may be localized or generalized.
- Spacing may be unilateral or bilateral.
- Spacing between two permanent maxillary central incisors in the midline is often referred to as midline diastema.

Diagnosis of Class I Malocclusion with Spacing

For diagnosis of this condition, a thorough examination should be supplemented with routine orthodontic diagnostic aids such as orthodontic study models to evaluate arch length—tooth material discrepancy and radiographic examination to rule out bony pathologies and unerupted teeth in the jaws.

Treatment of Class I Malocclusion with Spacing

I. Removal of the etiologic causes

III. Treatment of Class I malocclusion with spacing by using removable Orthodontic appliances, Simple removable orthodontic appliance with labial Bow or finger springs may be used to close the spacing in the arch.

IV. Treatment of Class I malocclusion with spacing by using fixed orthodontic appliances Fixed orthodontic appliance can be used to close the spaces by employing any of the following active components:

- E-chain (short or long)
- Closed coil spring.
- Elastics
- Elastic thread

V. Treatment of Class I malocclusion with spacing by conservative approach.

In cases of minor spacing in the arch, conservative approach can also be employed using appropriately shade-matched composite resin restorations.

CHAPTER I / CLASS I - EARLY AGE

CROWDING

Crowding occurs where there is a discrepancy between the size of the teeth and the size of the arches. The elective extraction of teeth is one method of alleviating crowding. In a crowded arch, the loss of a permanent or deciduous tooth will result in the remaining teeth tilting or drifting into the space created. This tendency is greatest when the adjacent teeth are erupting.

Mild: 1-3mm **Moderate:** 4-6mm **Severe:** >7 mm

MILD CROWDING

If the patient is treated at an early age, the duration and complexity of treatment that is required at a later stage may be reduced. (Fig.3)

If mild crowding is present, the first step would be to utilize space which can be attained naturally by:

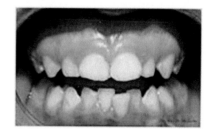

Fig 3

1. Leeway space (Fig.5)

2. Growth (growth increases arch length)

3. Primate space (between upper b & c, and lower c & d). (Fig.4)

4. Spacing in deciduous teeth.

5. The labial eruption of permanent upper centrals incisors.

If any of the above-mentioned points are missing/do not occur, this may lead to crowding.

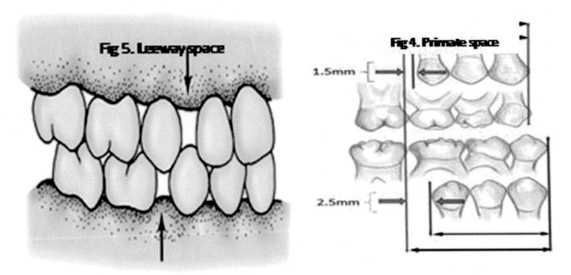

Fig 4. Primate space   Fig 5. Leeway space

How to relieve mild crowding?

1. Expansion: Expansion of the upper arch must be done early on, as the maxilla it completes growth at *8-9 years of age. (Fig. 6)*

- ○ Not a great amount of expansion is needed at this stage, just enough to create space.
- ○ It can be performed with a removable appliance and an expansion screw.
- ○ If expansion is done in normal conditions it can lead to scissor bite, therefore expansion should be done for 2mm only, so the cusp/fossa relationship is edge to edge and not exceeding this.
- ○ The lower arch will adapt to the upper after a while.
- ○ The removable appliance can be maintained as retention.

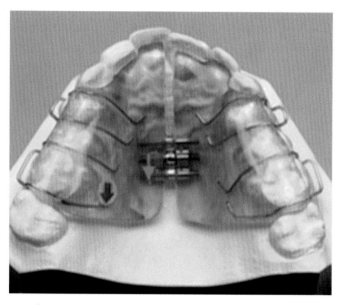

Fig 6. Removable appliance with expansion screw

2. Slicing of deciduous teeth mesially (never distally). (Fig. 7)

- ◦ This transfers leeway space anteriorly.

- ◦ To prevent the loss of the leeway space, a space maintainer must be placed to hold the molar in its position. (TPA or Nance in the upper, and lingual bar in lower). The leeway space will be consumed by the anterior crowding.

- ◦ For mild crowding slicing of the canines mesially can be done, to get 1-2mm of space and relieve the anterior crowding.

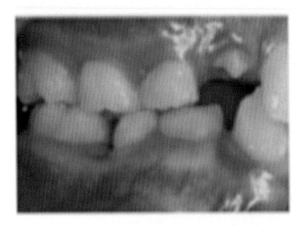 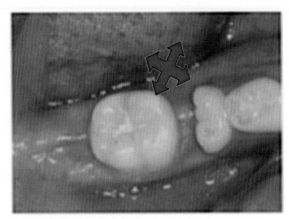

Fig 7. Slicing of primary teeth should be performed mesially, not distally.

3. Proclination to gain space.

- ◦ 1-2mm of proclination to increase overjet by 3 and 4mm. (1mm of proclination gives 2 mm of arch perimeter.)
- ◦ A Hawley appliance with a recurve spring can be used to push the 4 anterior teeth. **(Ironing effect)**. (Fig. 8)
- ◦ 1 degree of proclination will give less than 1mm. (0.8-0.9 increase in arch perimeter).
- ◦ If there is no compliance from the patient, a 2x4 can be used.
- ◦ Utility arches can be used. These will procline the anterior teeth and tip the molars distally, therefore anchorage must be reinforced with a TPA. To prevent opening of the bite, the wire should be bent to slightly extrude the incisors.

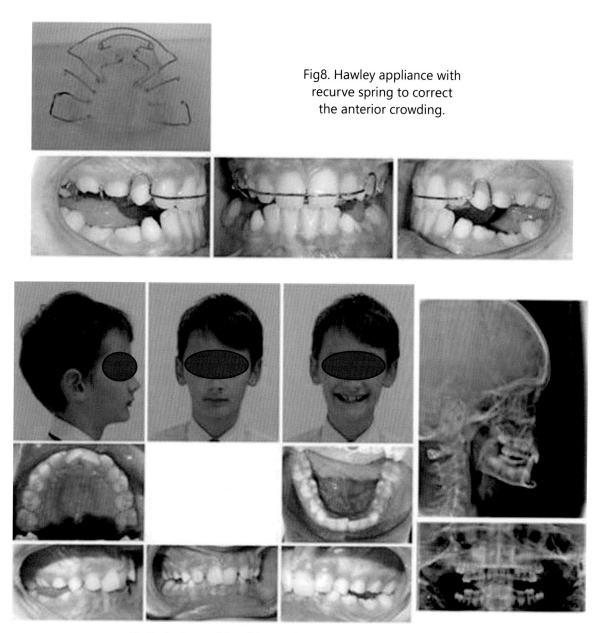

Fig8. Hawley appliance with recurve spring to correct the anterior crowding.

Fig9. Patient with mild anterior crowding: before treatment

Hawley appliance with recurve for mild crowding

MODERATE CROWDING

- Moderate crowding will require both expansion and proclination.
- Proclination can be done with a recurve spring.
- Slicing of the E's mesially to make use of the leeway space.
- Both mild and moderate crowding can be done with removable appliance.

SEVERE CROWDING

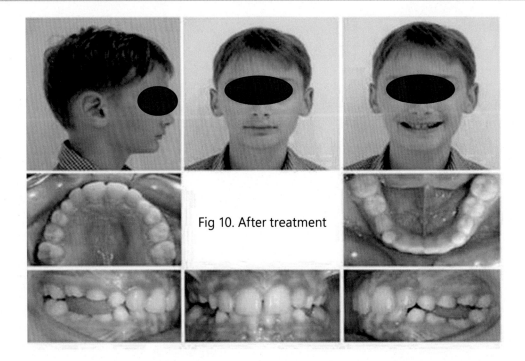

Fig 10. After treatment

- The serial extraction process starts at the age of 8.5 – 9 years. (Fig. 11)
- The prescribed order is C, D,4, E in all quadrants
  - Upper and lower must be done together.
- For very severe crowding with serial extraction, maximum anchorage may be required.

- ◦ Upper TPA
- ◦ Lower lingual arch
- ▪ Extraction of primary teeth should be performed when the permanent roots are $^2/_3$ to ¾ formed.

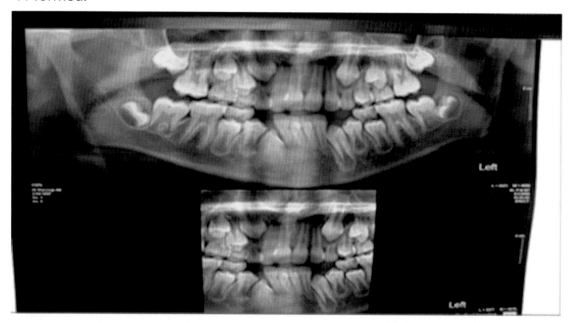

Fig 11. OPG showing severe crowding.

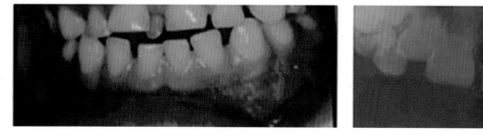

Fig 12. Supernumerary teeth should be removed immediately, even in the primary dentition.

ANTERIOR OPEN BITE WITH MILD CROWDING

- There is always a cause with an open bite.
- The first thing to look at is habits. Ask the patient or ask the patient to show you. E.g., finger sucking etc. Also ask the patient how he is during resting.
- If there is no habit, think of tongue position and mouth breathing.
- Whatever the cause is, you can't start treatment without removing the habit. Either by habit breaker or reminder therapy.
- *Habit breaker should be present from 6 months to 1 year.*
- Stop habit then start treatment.
- If treated early, stopping the habit will reduce the need for treatment. Teeth will go back to the normal position when the habit is stopped. (Auto correction).
- Extrusion of the incisors will gain space. Therefore, an open bite with mild crowding can be corrected on its own. As teeth are still erupting therefore you gain space by this natural extrusion.
- *Plan B-* if there is no autocorrection, 2x4 appliance should be used. This can be done using utility arch with an extrusion bend. The molar will tip mesially. To avoid this, anchorage is required (TPA).
- Anchorage is always required when using a utility arch. A force placed on anterior teeth will result in posterior forces and movement if anchorage is not enforced.
- Never correct open bite without correction of the AP dimension first. If OJ is insufficient, it will lead to an edge-to-edge bite, and further correction of the OB will not be possible.
- Over correction is needed to reduce relapse.

- Removable appliances can also be used for extrusion (e.g., Ismail's appliance):

  - Retention would be – Adams clasp between D.E and posterior bite plate. (Posterior bite plate here will intrude molars, hence closing the bite)
  - Recurved spring to move teeth vertically to close the open bite and/or horizontally to correct mild crowding if present.

ANTERIOR OPEN BITE WITH MODERATE CROWDING

- Break the habit and then reevaluate.
- If it didn't resolve on its own, then slicing or expansion
- If it does not, use a 2x4 utility arch and TPA with extrusion forces on the anterior teeth.

ANTERIOR OPEN BITE WITH SEVERE CROWDING

- Break the habit then proceed with serial extraction.
- If it is very severe, serial extraction and TPA to prevent the 6s from mesialization.

POSTERIOR OPEN BITE WITH MILD CROWDING

- Look for the cause, could be because of the tongue or the thumb, myofunctional appliances, such as Frankel or MyoBrace, can be used to block the effect of the tongue on the teeth.
- Myofunctional treatment is very important at an early age.
- Functional appliance must be used and not habit breaker.

DEEPBITE

DEEP BITE WITHOUT CROWDING

- Treatment with anterior bite plate will allow for extrusion of posterior teeth, and slight intrusion of anterior teeth.
- URA: A Hawley appliance with an anterior bite plate can be used. (Fig. 13)
- Fixed anterior bite plate with bands on U6`s. (Fig. 14)

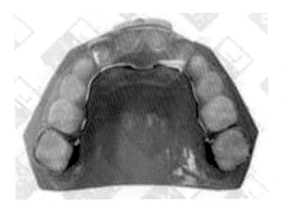

Fig13.URA anterior bite plate

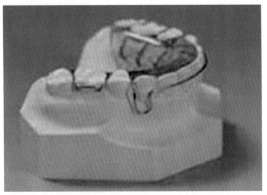

Fig14.Fixed anterior bite plate

DEEP BITE WITH MILD & MODERATE CROWDING

- Treatment must include slight expansion to create more space and proclination which opens the bite.
- When you procline the upper the lower will follow.
- Slight proclination will help when intruding teeth, as to not worsen the crowding.
- Anterior bite plate used in mild crowding.
- Expansion, slicing, proclination etc. can also be used as mentioned earlier.

DEEP BITE WITH SEVERE CROWDING

- Treat the deep bite first as above then proceed with serial extraction.
- Extraction deepens the bite.
- After each step you have to re-evaluate.

CROSSBITE

ANTERIOR SINGLE TOOTH

- Every crossbite must be treated ASAP (as soon as possible).
- Treatment can be done with removable or fixed appliances.
- A Z-spring, Adams clasp and I-clasp between D + E is a good configuration.
- The case below show a single tooth cross bite resulting in a traumatic and gingival recession. An URA appliance with posterior bite plate and Z-spring was used for correction of the cross bite and results in the natural resolution of the gingival recession of the 41. (Fig 15)

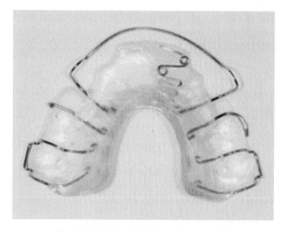

Fig15. URA with Z spring on 11, posterior bite plate and Hawley with retention Adams clasps and I clasp.

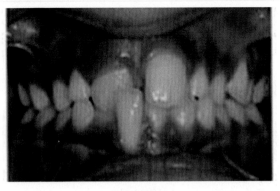
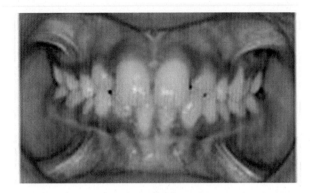

BEFORE   AFTER

- If overbite is more than 2mm, a posterior bite plate will be needed. Don't keep it for a long time, as soon as you jump the occlusion, remove it to prevent creation of a deep bite.
- If OB is less than 2 mm, a posterior bite plane is not required due to the freeway space.
- Labial bow placed to prevent teeth from rotating while we push the tooth.

MULTIPLE TEETH

- Hawley appliance is used with recurved spring palatally and labial bow.
- We can also use an expansion screw anteriorly to push the whole anterior segment forward.

ANTERIOR CROSSBITE WITH MILD CROWDING

- Proclination will create space, if not enough, expansion will be needed.
- (2x4 can also correct the crossbite, utility arch, TPA etc.)
- If all the crowding is concentrated in the centrals and there's no space for it to go out.
- Check crossbite, to open the bite place posterior bite raisers.
- In order to maintain molar relationship and position always reinforce anchorage. (TPA)

ANTERIOR CROSSBITE WITH MODERATE CROWDING

- Solve the cross bite by pushing the anterior teeth forward. This will create space to relieve the crowding and correct the cross bite. If space is still deficient, slicing of the C's will be needed.

ANTERIOR CROSSBITE WITH SEVERE CROWDING

- Extract the C's and procline the anterior teeth.
- Solve the crossbite and then start serial extraction.

POSTERIOR CROSSBITE

- Posterior bite planes can be used to correct posterior crossbites.
- Anterior bite plate should be used to jump the occlusion for scissor bites.
- Expansion must be done.
- Bilateral or Unilateral cross bites may be present.
- Unilateral can be true or false.
- **True:** is when the patient opens and closes the midline is on, so it's a dental crossbite.
- **False:** when the patient opens the midline is on, when he closes the midline is off, meaning there is a functional shift. (Forced bite)
- True unilateral cross bites require expansion on the affected side only. (Removable appliance with an expansion screw or quadhelix.)
- False unilateral cross bites require bilaterally expansion with a removable appliance with an expansion screw, with posterior bite plate if needed. (To dis-occlude and allow movement of teeth) Or a fixed bonded hyrax.
- Bilateral: expand both sides.

- Treated by either removable appliance or bonded hyrax. And in bilateral, midlines are on, there is no shift.
- Whatever appliance you use, leave it for at least 6 months for retention.

POSTERIOR CROSSBITE WITH MILD CROWDING

- With mild crowding, any expansion would be favorable as you will gain more space.

POSTERIOR CROSSBITE WITH MODERATE CROWDING

- Use recurve spring with Hawley arch, cut the recurve spring into half for expansion, to relieve the crowding so the expansion will be in three directions to gain space and relieve crowding.

POSTERIOR CROSSBITE WITH SEVERE CROWDING

- Expand first then reevaluate if you need to go for serial extraction after the expansion.

ANTERIOR CROSSBITE WITH DEEPBITE

- Deep bite with cross bite, also expand anteriorly by proclination it will cause flaring of the teeth and fix the deep bite.
- First fix the anterior crossbite (ASAP) (AP) then the Deep bite. (Vertical).
  - Start with a posterior bite plane, jump the crossbite, then remove the posterior bite plane.
  - Proclination to correct the cross bite will reduce the deep bite. An anterior bite plane may be required if the deep bite persists after correction of anterior cross bite.

POSTERIOR CROSSBITE WITH DEEPBITE

- Why do we use posterior bite plane with posterior crossbite?
  - To remove the occlusion of teeth and allow expansion without shifting. In a deep bite with post. cross bite, it is better to use the anterior bite plane especially with URA to reduce the deep bite and to open occlusion posteriorly.

- In cases of using removable appl. in mixed dentition. Expansion will be 1 turn per week, which will equal 1mm per month. (0.25mm per week). Fixed bonded hyrax could be used with one turn every day. (Limited use because it increases the deep bite because of posterior bite plane)

- For permanent banded hyrax, with deep bite and posterior crossbite, you will need anterior bite plane. The expansion will correct the deep bite then revaluate and anterior bite plane in the UR app. The deep bite could be corrected later with 2x4

- In the mixed dentition: If its dental we go for quadhelix, if skeletal, we use a banded hyrax. (bonded hyrax may deepen the bite)

POSTERIOR CROSSBITE WITH OPENBITE

- Open bite is associated with posterior crossbite.
- Mostly it is due to habit. (99.9%) Thumb sucking, and tongue thrusting removes the force to resist the lateral force on the palate, leading to collapse of the upper arch.
- All crossbites need to be corrected to have group function.
- Any expansion will open the bite more anteriorly.
- Expansion first is carried at the early age, but prior to that, the habit must be stopped first by a habit breaker. It may be possible that the appliance used for expansions can be designed to help stopping the habit.
- Posterior bite plate can be added along with the expansion to help in deepening the bite.
- Whether it's unilateral or bilateral, with or without shift. Place a posterior bite plate.
- If you have bilateral crossbite, you can also use the bonded hyrax.

- If the open bite is not corrected by itself after stopping the habit, then use 2+4 with TPA.
- Never close the open bite if you don't have enough overjet. It will lead to edge-to-edge bite. Opposite is for deep bite; you must get rid of the deep bite and then reduce overjet.
- Open bite: Correct AP (increase OJ) then Vertical (close the bite)
- Deep bite: Correct Vertical (open the bite) then AP (correct the OJ)
- Rx: stop the habit by tongue crib + quadhelix or tongue crib + W arch, we can use these devices with 2+4 with utility arch to correct the open bite anteriorly.

POSTERIOR CROSSBITE WITH OPENBITE + MILD/MODERATE CROWDING

- It will be solved by gaining space from expansion or extrusion.

  Stop the habit first!

  The expansion & extrusion as mentioned above.

POSTERIOR CROSSBITE WITH OPENBITE + SEVERE CROWDING

- Always stop the habit first then start the treatment.
- Next step expansion
- Extraction might be needed after finishing the expansion it's favorable as extraction deepens the bite.

All the above malocclusions that are associated with muscle function abnormality and/or some habitual mouth breathing at an early age and even in mid mixed dentition can be managed by myofunctional appliances. At an early age, these appliances can solve a lot of malocclusion problems or at least show big improvement.

CHAPTER II / CLASS I - MIDDLE AGE

CROWDING

MILD CROWDING

- Expansion can be performed.
- Proclination with removable and recurve spring or 2x4 appliance.
- Slicing from C`s to the E's
- Maintain the leeway space with TPA and lower lingual arch.

MODERATE CROWDING

- 2x4 appliance for proclination plus slicing
- If you have anterior crowding and the 4's aren't erupted, slice the C's, if the 4's are erupted slice the Es.
- If you want to use a removable appliance, same as previous, removable with recurve spring and expansion screw for little expansion if needed to gain space.

SEVERE CROWDING

- You can perform extractions.
- At this stage the most important thing is to evaluate the position of the canine and it`s inclination clinically and radiographically
- Extraction of c's, if required, should be performed in in all quadrants, not in only one arch or one side
- In severe crowding you need to determine if premolar extractions will be enough to relieve the crowding, if not, a space maintainer will be required.
- If the patient in middle age goes through serial extraction. To prevent space closure and loss of space, place a TPA/ lingual arch.

OPENBITE

ANTERIOR OPEN BITE AND CROWDING

- Stop the habit either by habit breaker or motivation. (Fig.16)
- If there is no spontaneous improvement, a 2x4 appliance with utility arch can be used to relieve the crowding (mild and moderate crowding)
- A habit breaker can also act as an anchorage reinforcement.
- The length of the tongue crib for tongue thrusting should be at the level of the cingulum of the lower incisors (without touching them)
- Severe crowding, serial extraction to be done.

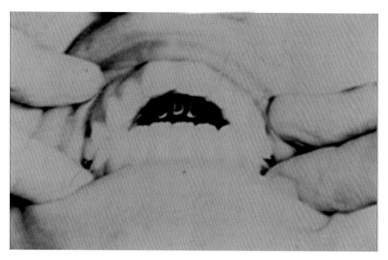

Fig16. Fixed habit breaker tongue grip.

POSTERIOR OPEN BITE AND CROWDING

- Frankel or myofunctional appliances can be used to obtain soft tissue balance

DEEPBITE

- ABP using either fixed or removable appliance
- Determine whether the deep bite is because of anterior extrusion or posterior intrusion. How? By looking at the smile line and the curve of spee.
- If you have a gummy smile then you need to do anterior intrusion with 2x4 appliance, and a utility arch with intrusion bend.
- Look at the curve of spee, if it is accentuated use a 2x4 appliance with a fixed anterior bite plane to get benefit of anterior bite plain at least 3months then bonding lower arch and a reverse-curve of spee if all premolars are erupted in the lower arch where you will extrude the posterior and slightly intrude the lower incisors.
- The fixed ABP will act as an anchorage for the 2x4 utility arch, to intrusion the upper anteriors and ABP help intrusion of lower incisors, and extrusion of posterior teeth.

DEEPBITE WITH MILD & MODERATE CROWDING

- Space is required to correct deep bites.
- **Mild:** proclination will help to reduce the deep bite and correct the mild crowding then evaluate anterior bite plate might be needed for intrusion
- **Moderate:** proclination with slight slicing from the deciduous (C's) and wait for full permanent then revaluate
- Anterior bite plate can be placed to help correct the deep bite.
- Factors that lead to opening of the bite:

  1) Extrusion of posterior teeth

  2) Intrusion of anterior teeth

  3) Proclination of anterior teeth

- Don't remove bite plate without placing fixed appliance on the lower to avoid relapse.
- The lower dentition should not be bonded at once with the anterior bite plate, as it will prevent the natural extrusion of the, if you brace the lower immediately, the molars will be prevented from erupting.

DEEPBITE WITH SEVERE CROWDING

- Extraction must be done but it will increase the deep bite.
- So first start by opening the bite, follow the same sequence with ABP then continue treatment like a normal bite patient.
- Extraction done after treating the deep bite. (Theoretically takes 3-6 months, but clinically depends on patient to patient).

- Minimum of 3 months for use of ABP before bonding the lower.
- Anterior bite plate must open the bite a minimum of 5 mm to open the bite. This will activate the muscle. If it's less than 5mm there will be no extrusion of the posterior teeth. (To overcome the leeway space)

CROSSBITE

ANTERIOR CROSSBITE WITH CROWDING (MILD + MODERATE)

- >2mm posterior bite plate
- Use 2x4 appliance with utility arch with internal coil.
- Posterior bite raisers are used if needed. >2mm

We can use URA with recurve spring & PBP procline anterior teeth and correct crowding. (Fig. 17)

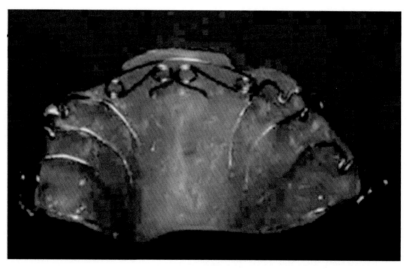

Fig17. URA with recurve spring Adams clasp on molars
and premolars with posterior bite plate (PBP).

- **Mild:** Procline upper teeth
- **Moderate:** Procline and slice the deciduous (C's)
- **Severe:** extraction might be needed.
- Anterior cross bite with deep bite posterior bite plain is a must in URA a bite raiser in fix then remove the bites after jumping the occlusion immediately.

POSTERIOR CROSSBITE

- If its true unilateral, use quadhelix only activate the arm of the cross-bite area, or removable the expansion screw is situated only on cross bite area and acrylic also should be cut in this region only always use PBP with it.
- Never use hyrax in true unilateral posterior crossbite because it leads to scissor bite on the correct side.
- If it's false unilateral diagnosed by shifting in mid line and bilateral – quadhelix or hyrax. (Fig.18 and Fig 19)
- If associated with crowding mild, moderate or severe after correction post cross bite you gain space you evaluate then in severe extract after expand.

POSTERIOR CROSSBITE WITH DEEPBITE

- ABP plus expand the quadhelix (goshgarian) arms or soldered arms to cause expansion.
- After correcting everything and evaluating decide if extraction if needed with present of crowding.
- Never extract before correcting the deep bite and the cross bite.
- Expansion helps to reduce the deep bite, never use PBP. Try not to use the bonded hyrax.
- Anterior bite plain may be sometimes used to reduce the deep bite if it still exists and at same time it holds the expansion previously done by the hyrax.

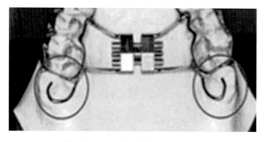

Fig18. Banded hyrax RPE.

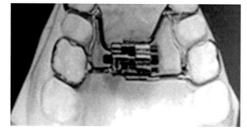

Fig19. Banded hyrax RPE.

POSTERIOR CROSSBITE WITH OPENBITE & WITH MILD, MODERATE AND SEVERE CROWDING

- Get rid of the habit, then expand with hyrax or quadhelix as above. These devices might also be used to stop the habit. We can use fixed and removable appliance (Ismail device) (fig.20) using an upper removable appliance with Labial to extrude the anterior centrals.
- Expansion then extraction, never do the opposite.

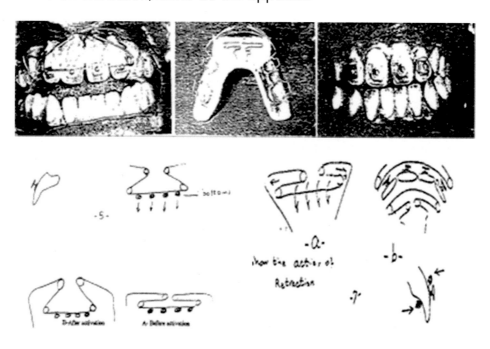

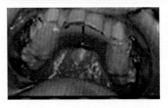

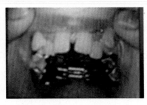

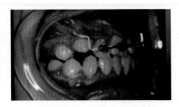

URA expansion screw PBP   Fix Hyrax for expansion.   Anterior expansion with 2x4 utility arch

SPACING

Spacing is due to either congenital missing teeth or tooth size arch length discrepancy. (fig.21a, b)

- Congenital missing teeth
- Missing upper lateral

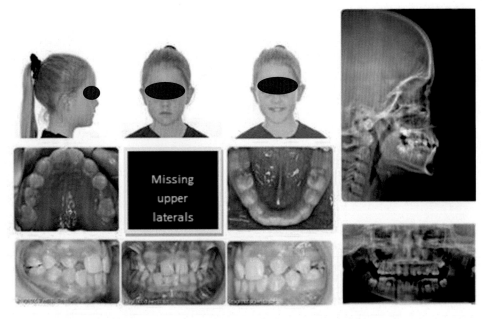

Fig21a) Missing upper laterals at a young age should be treated by canine substitution with mesial movement of the molars

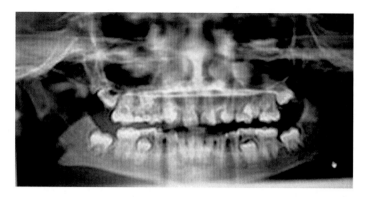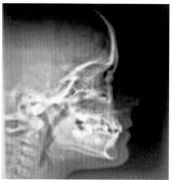

Fig21b) OPG and lateral cephalogram showing the missing teeth and patient profile which can accept the canine substitution.

CHAPTER III / CLASS I – ADULT

CROWDING

MILD CROWDING

- Use of fixed appliance
- Space can be gained by proclination if the profile allows, or correction of arch form.
- Bolton discrepancy will be seen.
- IPR could be sufficient. Last decision if no Bolton U&L IPR
- Clear aligner treatment can also be performed.

MODERATE CROWDING

- Widening of the arch
- Increase OJ if profile allows.
- Start non-extraction. Never perform IPR before making the extraction decision
- If you retract 1 mm you need 2 mm space. Therefore, if you procline 1mm, you gain 2mm.
- In Class I, premolar extractions should be performed in both Upper and lower arches.
- Extraction of a lower central is possible if the lower Bolton excess exceeds 4mm.
- Clear aligner treatment can also be performed.

SEVERE CROWDING

- Extraction 4 premolars if all teeth are sound) with fixed U&L appliances. (Fig.22)
- Always CL I sever crowding in extraction case has to be four quadrant in order to maintain the class one molar and canine relationship (not necessary the premolars it depend on the case and/or present or absent of dental caries.

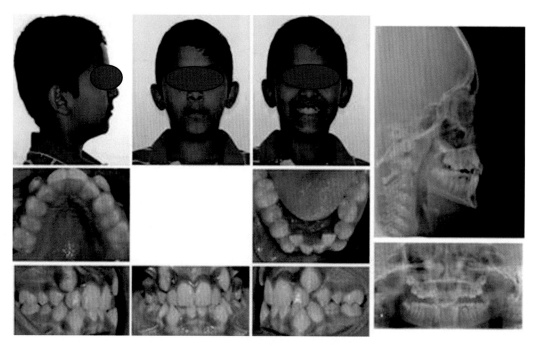

Fig.22. Very severe crowding treated with extraction of the four premolars.

OPENBITE

- ***When closing the open bite. know how severe it is & stop any habits***
- Types of closure: reciprocal. Upper and lower fixed appliance with anterior box intermaxillary elastics.
- Extrusion of the upper anterior teeth is mostly done. As the lower is limited by the bone and tissue.

- If there is limited incisal display on smiling, then more extrusion of the upper anterior teeth is required.
- Excessive extrusion of lower anteriors can cause recession. Always check alveolar bone and gingiva. Check periodontal condition before choosing what to extrude.
- In cases where you can't extrude anterior teeth, intrude posterior teeth. (6 and 7)
- Open bite will always have an underlying factor, therefore always know the cause, usually either thumb sucking or tongue thrusting.
- If the thumb sucking or tongue thrusting habits persist with growth, skeletal changes will occur.
- If no habit is detected, size or position of the tongue may be the cause.
- If a gummy smile is present, don't extrude upper anteriors, but intrude posterior. If you want to extrude lower anterior, use a heavy wire on upper arch and lighter wire on lower arch.
- Correction of OJ must be done prior to closure of the open bite. Extrusion bends on the anterior teeth will correct the OB as well.
- Fixed in upper and lower will be used, then decide if box elastics will be sufficient or extrusion bend will be needed.
- Heavy wire can be placed in the lower arch and lighter wire in the upper arch if you want to extrude the uppers.

ANTERIOR OPENBITE WITH SEVERE CROWDING

- Treat the cause first.
- Extract to relieve crowding and to deepen bite.
- TADs can be used to intrude molars. 4 or 6 TADs placed buccally and palatally with elastic chain crossing the occlusal surfaces of both sides.
- Buccal TADs with TPA can also be used to intrude the posterior teeth. The loop in TPA should face anteriorly and be 4-5mm away from the palate. The TPA will prevent buccal tipping during intrusion.

DEEPBITE

DEEPBITE AND CROWDING

RESOLVE DEEP BITE FIRST

Fixed appliances U&L

- For adults, it is preferred to use ABP.
- Crowding and deep bite correction requires space.
- Slight proclination, if possible, will relieve mild crowding and help mitigate the deep bite.
- If you have a deep bite because of the upper anterior teeth then you need to focus on that and intrude. this can be checked by the incisal display on smiling.
- If it`s because of the lower, and the incisal display on smiling is normal, check the curve of spee, and focus on treating the lower.
- In both cases know the cause.
- Extrude posterior teeth to open space if needed.
- **ABP** – and intermaxillary elastics to extrude the molars.
- **Accentuated Curve of Spee** – extrusion of premolar area.
- **Turbo** – bracket bonded on lingual side, to open the bite posteriorly.
  - Problem is that all the force is located on the 2 centrals.
  - Do not use bite raisers/turbos on any tooth you want to move.
- Always bond the 7`s in deep bite cases especially the lower.
- Sometimes you would need to use posterior box intermaxillary elastics to extrude the upper and lower teeth. Must be done on light wires to hasten the process. (With the anterior bite plate)
- **Treat the deep bite first, then correct the crowding like mentioned above.**

- In deep bite, hypodivergent adults (who usually have severe bruxism and grinding), it is very difficult to move teeth and close the spaces.

- With mild crowding, IPR can be performed to minimize proclination.

- Moderate crowding requires the same as above, but we need stripping U&L

- Try to avoid extraction of lower central with Bolton in deep bite unless we are sure of correction of deep bite, and this is the only choice

- Severe crowding after correction of deep bite: extraction is required.

- If we want to relieve the deep bite completely after all the steps above and using RCoS wires. TAD`s placed buccally can be used for intrusion of upper centrals or intrusion of lower centrals. (Fig. 25a, b)

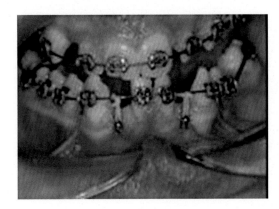 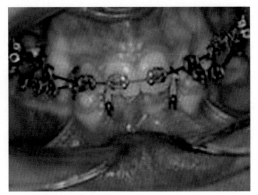

Fig.25b
TAD`s for intrusion upper centrals because of the deep bite caused by the extrusion of the upper centrals.

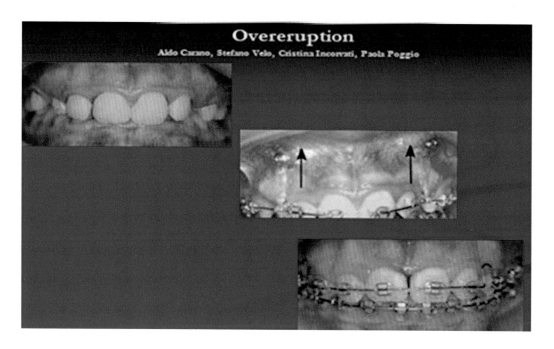

Fig.25a
TAD`s for intrusion of lower centrals because of the deep bite from the lower teeth

CROSSBITE

ANTERIOR CROSSBITE WITH CROWDING

- Fixed upper and lower.
- If you need to open the bite, use posterior bite raisers to open the bite. (If more than 2mm)
- **Mild & moderate:** by correcting the crossbite you will gain space. might strip.
- **Severe:** alignment and proclination of anterior teeth, deal with the cross bite first and then go to crowding. extraction later

POSTERIOR CROSSBITE WITH CROWDING

- If it is true unilateral, use quadhelix in mild cases or archwire and cross elastics.
- If it is false unilateral, hyrax or quadhelix.
- Severe bilateral: hyrax or MARPE. Skeletal expansion will be needed not just dental expansion.
- **TAD** must be placed as close as possible to the center of the palate as the bone thickness of the palate is thicker whereas it is too thin laterally.
- Always keep the device of expansion at least 6months after finishing the expansion.
- If the posterior cross bite is minimal with mild crowding, we can use aligners which can help in little posterior expansion and correction of the crowding with or without IPR.

POSTERIOR CROSSBITE WITH ANTERIOR OPENBITE

- Treat crossbite first, place Hyrax.
- Hyrax will prevent the habit and will improve mouth breathing.
- Bonded (or hyrax with posterior bite plane) hyrax will help the open bite as it will intrude posterior teeth as well.
- Compliance is needed as it is uncomfortable for adults.
- Intrude posterior teeth.
- Don't close the bite if you feel the teeth will end in cross bite or edge to edge, first procline teeth and correct the AP, then close the open bite. (Transverse, AP then Vertical)
- Try to avoid the use of posterior cross elastics in open bite cases to correct the cross bite as it will extrude posterior teeth more, thus opening the bite. (It is better used in cases requiring extrusion of posterior teeth). TAD can be inserted during between premolar and molars buccally after the expansion with the same device to intrude posteriorly
- In very severe cases – surgery is needed. (After we use TAD to intrude post. teeth to close the ant open bite without any result)

CROSSBITE WITH DEEP BITE

- Expansion will help reduce the deep bite.
- When you expand you gain space.
- Treat cross bite first, then deep bite.
- Don't extract before expansion and correction of deep bite.
- Use fixed anterior bite plain with your fixed appliance if the deep bite still exists after the expansion. Always check which arch needs correction by looking at incisal display on smiling.
- If the posterior cross bite is mild, correction by arch wire and cross elastics can be used. It will also help to extrude molars and reduce the ant. deepbite.
- Always keep the expander device in for 6 months for retention, or until you reach a heavy wire in upper arch. Widen the archwire to compensate for relapse.

SPACING

When we have generalized spacing because of the difference between arch length and tooth size we must maintain the arch length by making a stop (omega) mesial to molar tube to prevent any collapse in the arch while we are pulling the individual teeth mesially to close the spaces. When the only space remaining is mesial to the molars, remove the stop, ligate 5-5, and mesialize the molars by elastic power chain.

Any time we want to prevent mesial drift of the molars or/and increase anchorage, we can use the omega stop mesial to the molar tube.

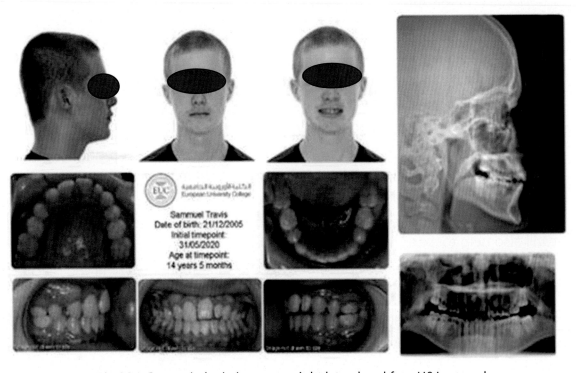

(Fig 26a) Congenital missing upper right lateral and four U&L second premolars with retained second primary molar (E's)

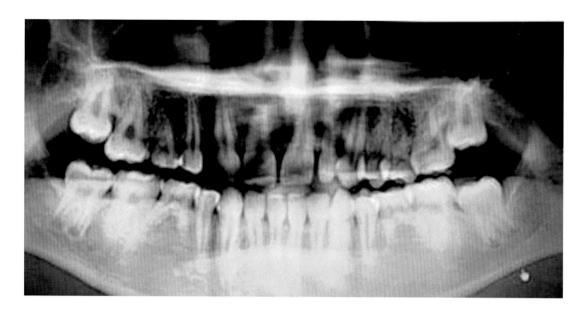

(Fig.26b) There is no root resorption of the Es so we maintain them and solve the missing lateral by opening the space for implant or canine substitution, but space will remain posteriorly because no mesial movement could be done for the molars because of the presence of E's.

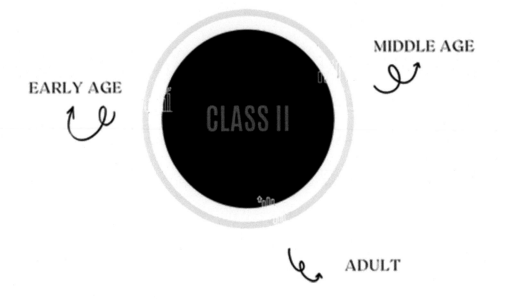

EARLY AGE

MIDDLE AGE

ADULT

CLASS II

Treatment of class II malocclusion differs from that of class I malocclusion in having the added complication of anteroposterior dental arch discrepancy along with crowding, rotations, etc. Therefore, in addition to the possible necessity of correcting crowding and irregularity of the teeth and any local anomalies, one of the main objectives in class II malocclusion treatment is the correction of the anteroposterior dental arch relationship.

ETIOLOGICAL FACTORS OF CLASS II MALOCCLUSION

Etiological factors causing Angle's class II malocclusion are categorized into the following three factors:

I. Prenatal factors

1. **Genetic and congenital:** Studies done on parents and children having the same type of malocclusion indicates that the facial dimensions are principally determined by heredity through genes. Hence, the dimensions of the basal bones which can contribute to skeletal class II malocclusion can be inherited.

2. **Teratogenesis:** Administration of certain drugs during pregnancy has a potential of yielding abnormal development of arches leading to class II malocclusion. Such drugs are referred to as teratogens.

3. **Irradiation:** Irradiation therapy during fetal life can also be a causative factor for class II malocclusion.

4. **Intrauterine fetal posture:** Abnormal posture of the fetus such as hands across the face is found to affect mandibular growth.

II. Natal factors

Improper forceps application during delivery can lead to condylar damage/fracture causing internal haemorrhage into the joint area. TMJ can get ankylosed or fibrosed later, leading to underdevelopment of the mandible.

III. Postnatal factors.

Certain conditions that can influence the normal development of the craniofacial skeleton are:

- Traumatic injuries during play
- Long-term irradiation therapy
- Oral habits such as thumb sucking
- Congenitally missing teeth
- Anomalies in the shape of teeth.

TREATMENT OF CLASS II DIVISION 1 MALOCCLUSION

The objective of treatment in patients with Angle's class II division 1 malocclusion includes:

_ Relief of crowding and local irregularities

_ Reduction of incisal overbite

_ Reduction of incisal overjet

_ Correction of class II relationship of the buccal teeth.

Management of class II malocclusion

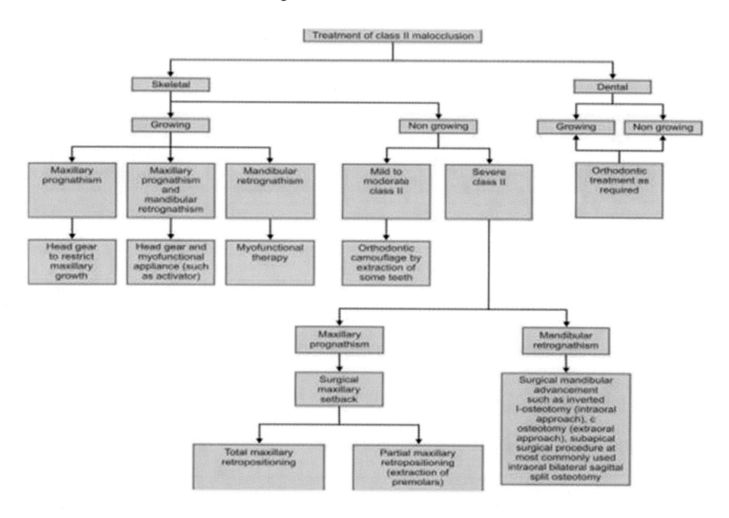

CHAPTER IV / CLASS II - EARLY AGE

CROWDING

NO CROWDING

- A little expansion can be done by removal appliance with an expansion screw.
- Expansion should cease at edge-to-edge position. Do not expand into a scissor bite.
- The patient will want to advance the mandible by autorotation to get cusp to fossa relationship.
- The expansion will be around 1-2mm.
- This will create auto functional appliance and advance the mandibular position and reduce overjet.

MILD CROWDING

- Do not treat patient with only deciduous dentition.
- Diagnose the case with eruption of centrals, laterals and 1st molars.
- Appliance you can use: Removable appliance with expansion screw.
- What will it do? Expand upper arch slightly. The patient will not be able to bite normally so will reposition his lower jaw to get better occlusion. In that way it will allow for forward growth of the mandible (natural functional appliance).

- This will also help with correction of crowding by creating space with expansion.
- Rx: Slicing of the C's and the D's can be done, or slight expansion with removable appliance.

MODERATE CROWDING

- Limited Expansion with removable appliance can be used, Recurve spring and Hawley arch may be placed.
- Limited Expansion will be required here, similar effect will happen as above (autorotation).
- Headgear can be used, especially if the maxillary incisors are severely proclined. Then 2x4 if needed

SEVERE CROWDING

- Correct to get class I (via limited expansion) then go with serial extraction.
- Start with upper then lower arch. (extraction)
- In the upper arch, extract what you need in the anterior segment then after extraction of premolar, go to lower arch.
- Check the canine position by X ray for decision of removing C`s.
- Always expansion before extraction!!!
- Headgear can be used to distalize upper molars and then re-evaluate for serial extraction.
- In every class II try to advance the mandible rather than distalizing the maxilla, only if you have obvious skeletal class II due to a prognathic maxilla, headgear can be used.

CROSSBITE

CROSSBITE WITH MILD & MODERATE CROWDING

- Expansion to correct crossbite. Gain space and relieve the mild or moderate crowding. We can do a little more expansion to let the mandible move forward for auto correction.
- More expansion will be needed compared to crowding cases alone. The mandible will then auto rotate.
- As always mentioned, determine if the cross bite is true unilateral or false with shift or bilateral.
- Again, expansion either by URA OR Quadhelix or bilateral Bonded hyrax

CROSSBITE WITH SEVERE CROWDING

- Expansion first then evaluate.
- Serial extraction might be needed here. Or only upper arch with the expansion first by same methods above.
- More space will be attained, auto correction etc.

OPENBITE

- Stop the habit by either reminder, habit breaker, etc.
- As this is a child, with the habit breaker alone and elimination of habit, the teeth are still extruding, therefore teeth will go back to normal by auto eruption.
- 2x4 might be used with tongue crib. **If the bite doesn't close on its own and patient doesn't stop the habit**. Everything in early age usually closes on its own when habit is eliminated.
- After the open bite is closed, we just deal with it like it's a normal class II.

- First, target the vertical problem (open bite) then AP (advance the mandible), unlike class I which is the opposite, because in class II we already have increased overjet.

- Class II open bite, you need expansion, add posterior bite plane, because even though you removed the cause, you need it to prevent reopening of the bite as expansion could open the bite.

OPENBITE WITH MILD CROWDING

- Space gained from expansion and extrusion of anterior teeth.

- With extrusion, more space will be gained, and with intrusion more space will be required.

- First step would be to deal with the vertical by stopping the habit then wait for auto eruption. If not, use 2x4 with the fixed habit breaker and utility arch with extrusion bend to extrude the rest of the anterior teeth resolving both the open bite and mild crowding.

- In using URA with habit breaker. Posterior bite plane can then be placed to intrude posterior teeth and close the bite. This will also free the patient from occlusion which will cause autorotation of the mandible.

- Head gear high pull sometimes it is helpful after little auto closure of the open bite & gain space and correction of the AP.

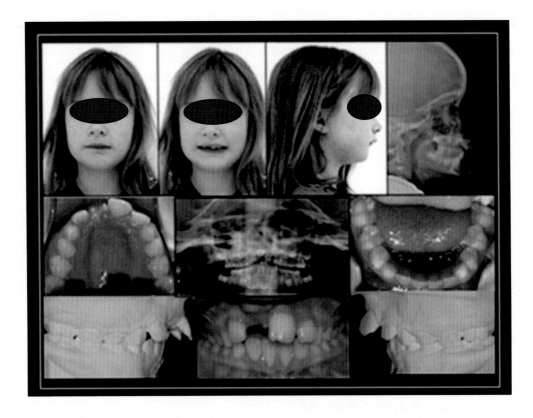

CL II patient with thumb sucking and impacted upper right central in a horizontal position.

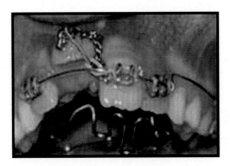

Before correction

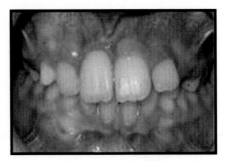

After correction

2x3 with Utility arch is used with extrusion bend on molar region to pull the impacted central 11 down with the anchorage to the molars by the habit breaker

Always keep in mind, that in class II and class III we have a higher chance of HAVING 2ND phase of treatment.

OPENBITE WITH MODERATE CROWDING

- Evaluate, if more space is required start with slicing after getting rid of the open after using fixed habit breaker and utility arch. Then we deal with the AP
- Again, high pull Head gear might be useful.

OPENBITE WITH SEVERE CROWDING

- Do as above then re-evaluate.
- Evaluate for extractions.
- Wait until 9.5 years of age then reevaluate for serial extraction.
- Myofunctional appliances can be used during early age (sometimes) and mixed dentition.
- Helps with abnormality in muscular function.

DEEPBITE

- **Add ABP with expansion using URA.**
- Same procedure as above.
- ABP can be inclined so the patient will protrude the mandible. Working as a functional appliance. (autorotate) (fig.27)
- If you don't want proclination of the lower, flat ABP to decrease the deep bite. It will touch the lower centrals. slight intrusion while extruding the molars to open the bite with limited expansion. (Fig.28a, b)
- **Division I:** ABP (inclined) + expansion
- **Division II:** ABP (inclined) + expansion + Recurve spring to procline upper incisors.

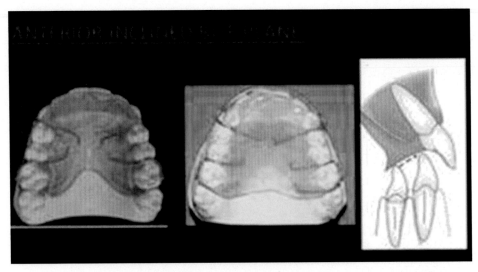

Fig27 Inclined anterior bit plate for decreasing the deep bite help in shifting the mandible forward and might create proclination to lower centrals

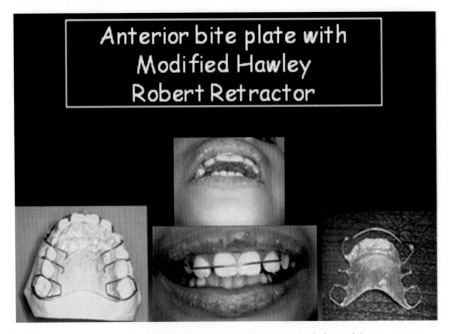

Fig. 28b CL II with Severe proclination and deep bite.
Phase 1: URA. To be prepared for second stage functional appliance

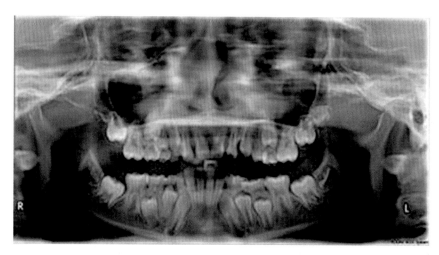

Cephalometric radiograph showing severe deep
bite and the OPG showing mixed dentition.

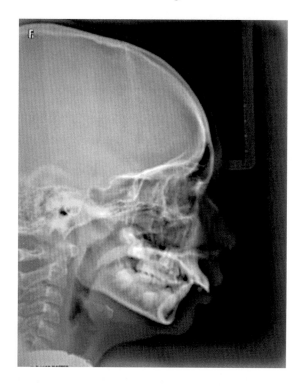

DEEP BITE AND ANTERIOR CROSSBITE

- Use a posterior bite plate and recurved spring to jump the occlusion anteriorly. Remove the PBP and continue proclination. This will improve deep bite.

- Distalization with a cervical pull head gear with 2x4 to correct cross bite and deep bite. The 2x4 should be a utility arch with internal helices.

DEEP BITE AND POSTERIOR CROSSBITE

- Almost always associated with a habit, therefore expand as much as possible.

- **Unilateral/True –** Quadhelix or removable appliance with Expansion screw cut the acrylic on the side of crossbite only.

- **Unilateral/ False –** Removable appliance with expansion screw in the middle with ABP, or bonded hyrax. The disadvantage is that it increases the deep bite because of the bite plane on the bonded hyrax. Thereafter expansion Hawley with anterior bite plain.

- **Bilateral -** Removable appliance with expansion screw in the middle, or bonded hyrax.

- Difference here is that overcorrection must be done for both.

- Correct crossbite then crowding then reevaluate if distalization is needed.

- For deep bites with posterior cross bites and mild and moderate crowding, we will gain space by expansion, which also gives the possibility for forward movement of the mandible.

- With severe crowding, reevaluate for extraction and/or phase 2.

- Cervical head gear with expansion can help in distalizing the molars and creating space.

IF YOU FAIL TO IMPROVE THE AP PREPARE THE PATIENT FOR THE SECOND PHASE WITH EXPANSION

CHAPTER V / CLASS II - MIDDLE AGE

- Perfect age for functional appliances in class II patients. (pre-peak)

- During the period of growth, you will get maximum benefits from functional appliance. (Fig.29a, b)

- For class II Division 2, first change it to class II Division 1, then use the functional appliance to advance the mandible. (Create enough OJ to advance the mandible).

- Done by recurve spring + expansion for 6 months to correct the retruded centrals.

- When the problem is in the maxilla, distalization can be done by headgear.

- If class II exists alone and expansion is needed, then twinblock can be used.

- It is preferable to bring the mandible forward rather than to bring maxilla back to maintain the airway. Therefore, the diagnosis should be accurate in order to determine if the problem is in the upper or lower arch.

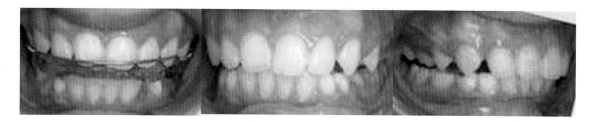

Fig.29a. Using functional appliance like a Bionator to correct the CL II div.1 with severe deep bite. Patient after 6 months of using the functional appliance.

Case 1: phase 2: Functional Appliance. (Post Tx.)

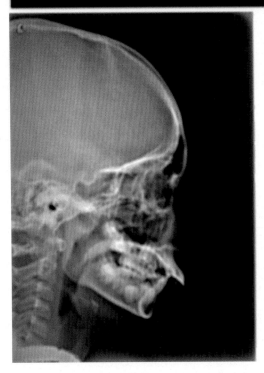

BEFORE

Fig.29b

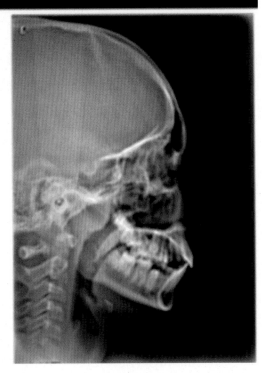

AFTER

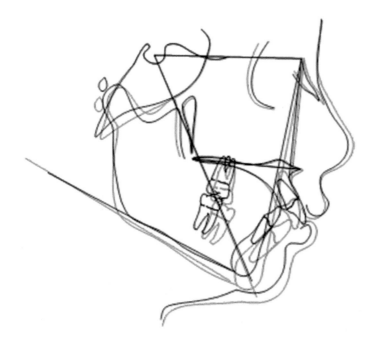

Superimposition of the ceph. Before and after the 2 phases of treatment:

URA first and functional appliance later

CROWDING

Crowding can be solved later, treat the most important factor first (the class II) to make use of growth. If this critical timepoint is missed, it will be too late to alter skeletal growth.

MILD AND MODERATE CROWDING

- If the patient arrives to the clinic during the critical period, treatment by functional appliance can be used.

- Twinblock can be used in this case, with expansion screw to advance the mandible and expand on the same time because any advancement may cause a cross bite posteriorly. When using a Bionator or monoblock, oblique trimming in the posterior area achieves the dental expansion. Thus, making the teeth tip buccally. Mesial trimming occlusally is also required to direct the lower molars to be in a more mesial position.

- If there is sufficient growth remaining, expansion can be started with a removable appliance followed immediately with a functional appliance.

- Mandible is retruded: Expansion with Quadhelix and then a functional appliance, then 2x4 appliance or full fixed appliance if premolars are already erupted after sagittal correction.

- Maxilla protruded: Expansion with Quadhelix then headgear then 2x4 appliance or complete fixed appliance for alignment. (Fig.30)

- If space is still needed for the crowding, we can slice the C`s.

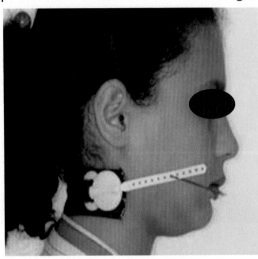

Fig.30. Using cervical pull head gear in CL II with deep bite

SEVERE CROWDING

- Treat AP first then deal with crowding in phase 2 with extraction, either serial or permanent.

- Calculate the space needed, there might be increased overjet and crowding.

- For example, if we have an OJ of 7mm and crowding of 10mm. that's 15mm required to fix both problems. If you start with extraction, you might relieve the crowding but there won't be enough space to fix the overjet. Therefore, AP must be corrected first, so in a case like this you won't look for an extra 5mm because of the overjet.

- If the problem is with the maxilla, and distalization is done (with HG), space is gained which may relieve the crowding. Therefore, re-evaluate first before deciding on extractions.

- Sometimes palatal TAD's can be used for distalization of the molars using a distal jet (fig.31)

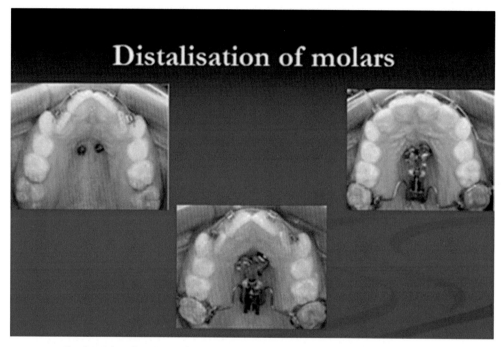

Fig 31. Distalization of molars with TAD's placed in the palatal area.

SEVERE CROWDING WITH SEVERE OVERJET

- Manage AP using functional appliance during this period to reduce overjet first then deal with the crowding. Extractions and the fixed appliance will likely also be required.

OPENBITE

- First stop the habit.
- Correct the open bite first then the overjet.

- Start with a tongue crib (treat the cause) and 2x4 appliance. Utility arch used here for extrusion after allowing 3 months to self-correct.
- Functional appliances are not indicated in open bites. A high pull headgear may be more appropriate.

OPENBITE WITH MILD & MODERATE CROWDING

- Habit breaker to treat the open bite, then treat the AP.
- Then high pull headgear with 2x4 fixed appliance or a Frankel appliance.

OPEN BITE WITH SEVERE CROWDING

- First habit breaker.
- Then extract (favorable, as extraction deepens the bite)
- If the crowding is in the upper only extract upper 4's only.
- If crowding is in the upper and lower, extract upper 4's and lower 5's.
- If there is severe crowding in the upper and lower anterior dentition, extract upper 4's and lower 4's. (extract near the crowded area), especially if full dentition or in very late mix dentition.

When there is openbite, whether IT'S class I or class II, first check if there is enough overjet. If overjet is not enough, treat AP then vertical.

DEEPBITE

- Functional appliance will open the bite. – You can trim the posterior occlusal surface to allow extrusion of the molars. (Fig.32a, b)
- Functional appliance will also procline the anteriors. Therefore, help with the deep bite and AP correction, re-evaluate.

- If the problem is from the maxilla, then use a cervical headgear. (Extrusion of molars and open the bite).

- It is better to advance the mandible than retract the maxilla.

- We can use a fixed inclined anterior bite plain to improve the deep bite.

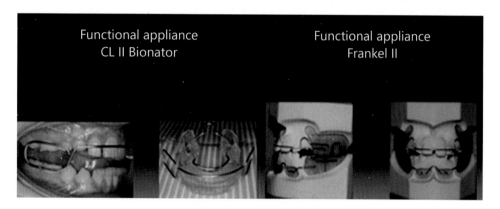

Fig.32a

DEEPBITE WITH MILD & MODERATE CROWDING

- Always treat the deep bite first, then treat the rest (AP and the crowding). Functional appliance is advantageous as it treats both AP & vertical simultaneously.

- We can treat the mild or moderate crowding later with fixed appliance.

- If we start with fixed appliance, a fixed anterior bite plane is required (preferably inclined especially if there is no lower proclination). Do not bond the lower arch immediately.

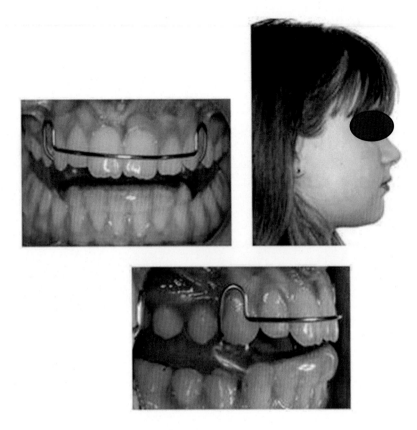

Fig.32b

- Effect of Rx by Functional appliance
- Allow the bite to plane enough time to be effective (minimum 3 months), and then bond the arches to improve crowding and for AP correction.
- If the problem is from the maxilla, we can start with a cervical head gear to help create space and correct the AP.

DEEPBITE WITH SEVERE CROWDING

- Treat deep bite first or simultaneously as above.
- Then treat the severe crowding with extraction of upper 4's using fixed appliance at this stage with fixed anterior bite plane. Make sure you manage the deep bite before or during extraction.

In class II Division II

- Convert to division 1 by inclined anterior bite plate, and with a 2x4 utility arch to procline upper anterior teeth.
- When it becomes CLII div. 1, then treat as above. One important thing to keep in mind try to avoid extraction especially in the lower. Three important things for CLII div.2: get rid of the deep bite, eliminate the pressure of the lower lip on the upper incisors (by increasing the vertical dimension) & obtaining a good inter incisor angle.

CROSSBITE

- Class II div.2 with anterior crossbite is not common. It may only be seen with Division II. This can be corrected with URA with Z springs, Adams, Hawley, PBP (fig.33a, b)

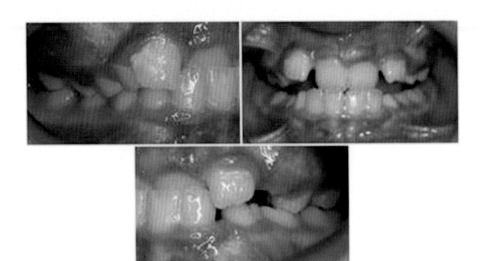

Fig33.a CLII div2 crossbite U centrals

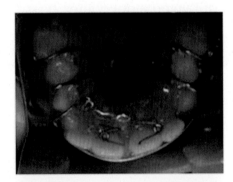

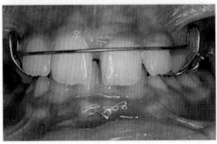

Fig 33.b URA   Z spring PBP Hawley Adams

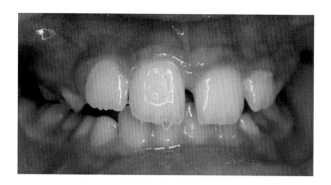

AFTER CORRECTION

Crossbite would be posteriorly with a class II and would most probably be due to habits, like thumb sucking. If so, get rid of the habit.Treat by expansion first, then go for functional appliance because we need more expansion. Treat transverse first then the AP.

- If we have bilateral crossbite it's better to expand with a hyrax because you will get skeletal expansion and at the same time create space.
- The hyrax allows for almost immediate expansion.
- It should stay for a minimum of 6 month to 1 year after expansion for retention.
- **Turns for expansion:**
  - Normal 1 turn/ day.
  - fast 2 turns/day
  - slow 1 turn/week (only for removable appliances)
- If the crossbite is not severe, and you're going to distalize then you can expand with the inner bow of the headgear.
- Quadhelix will give mostly dental effects used for unilateral, bilateral and anterior expansion. Advantage: you can control where to expand.
- Bonded – premolar not erupted.
- Banded – premolar erupted.

- Expansion will reduce the deep bite.
- Creates space.
- If the maxilla is tapered, and we expand with a hyrax the maxilla will remain tapered. So, it may be better to expand with a quadhelix.

CROSSBITE WITH MILD & MODERATE CROWDING

- Expand first to treat the crossbite and create space then advance the mandible or treat AP.

CROSSBITE WITH SEVERE CROWDING

- Expand first, keep the hyrax for retention, use functional appliance to reduce the overjet. Then re-evaluate if you need extractions.
- If extraction is needed, cut the hyrax at the premolar areas to extract the 4's, but keep it posteriorly for retention and anchorage. If we use quadhelix, expansion first then extract 4`s then fixed appliance.

CROSSBITE WITH OPENBITE & WITH THE CROWDING

- Expand with an expansion appliance acting as a habit breaker. That means eliminating the habit that caused the open bite and the cross bite at the same time.
- A tongue crib can be added to it.
- Expansion opens the bite therefore extrusion might be required.
- Then go for headgear or functional appliance.
- A bonded hyrax may be the best choice because of the posterior bite plate. This will help decrease the open bite by intrusion of the posterior teeth. We can then reevaluate the ant. Openbite. We keep the hyrax for retention while moving to fixed appliance to correct the CLII. A high pull head gear is beneficial especially when you have mild or moderate crowding. In severe crowding, extraction is often required.

- Start with expansion, try not to use bonded hyrax because of the posterior bite plate will deepen the bite.

- Expansion (with hyrax) here is favorable as it opens the bite and decreases the deep bite.

- If the quadhelix was used in the expansion the keep same device and start with fixed appliance.

- If expansion is not enough, then use an inclined anterior bite plane, to act as a functional appliance. And retain the expansion at the same time.

- Again, by expansion we gain space for resolving the mild and moderate crowding, but in severe crowding, although there is some space gain, extractions may be required.

- Remember always extract after expansion and deep bite resolution.

CHAPTER VI / CLASS II – ADULT

- Class II is either full-cusp (7mm) or half-cusp (3.5mm)

- ½ cusp (3.5mm) is class II but ¼ cusp isn't considered Cl II

- Very Severe class II (skeletal) with an unaesthetic profile: go for orthognathic surgery.

- Evaluate if patient is still growing or not.

- Then evaluate where the problem is from, to decide whether to distalize upper or advance the mandible.

- **Dentally deal with camouflage by:**

1. Mandible Advancement

2. Distalization

3. Extraction

   (Expansion will not let the Mandible to grow at this period)

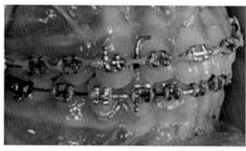

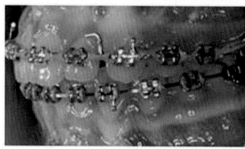

Fig.34 Rx by fix appliance with CLII elastics

1. Mandibular Advancement:

- If you need the effect of forward advancement after the patient has stopped growing and is in full permanent dentition, use either fixed functional appliance (forsus, Herbst) or class II elastics

- For full cusp class IIs, definitely use fixed functional appliance, if ½ cusp, elastics would work.

- CL II elastics (fig.34) and Herbst etc., acts to mesialize the lower dentition and distalize the upper, if there is no basal effect (skeletal effect), there will still be dentoalveolar effects.

- Herbst can correct overjet before crowding (used before alignment).

- Forsus is used after 6 to 12 months after alignment reaching heavy e.g., 0.019x0.025 SS.

- Lower incisor proclination is a side effect of forsus and elastics CLII so they can't be used with already proclined lower incisors.

For Forsus follow the points below after leveling and aligning:

- Heavy wires upper and lower (.019x.025 SS)
- Cinch behind the upper and lower 6s (directly behind the tube)
- It is essential to lace the lower teeth from 6 -6 (you can do upper as well, but lower is a must). If you don't lace the teeth, it would move canine and molar instead of the whole arch.
- Steel tie all the lower teeth and upper

2. Distalization:

- Carrier is also a distalizer.
- Carrier also needs compliance, as very heavy elastics must be used. (6-8 OZ)
- Carrier effects: Upper canine extrusion, Upper 1st molar rotation, lower incisor proclination, for this reason we use an essix in the lower arch which will somewhat prevent proclination of lower incisors.
- Headgear can't distalize more than half-cusp. Need compliance!
- Distalizer can be used with expander, to distalize molar and expand at the same time. Benefit or distal jet, pendulum ...etc.
- If it's not possible then extraction is also a choice.
- The distal jet also used for distalization. Has possibility of mesialization of anterior teeth proclination as well. Therefore, more favorable for class II div II.
- Never distalize molar and place TPA alone as a retainer after distalization but you can use palatal screw to hold the TPA.
- How can you stop the molar from going back mesially?
  - Distal jet (distalize or forsus to maintain) when you're pulling the teeth back.

- BeneFit system, minimum side effect, TADs placed in the middle of palate, with a heavy wire extending from the metal plate that is attached to the TADs to the palatal sheath on the molar bands. A screw is used to compress the coil and distalize the molar.

- The BeneFit system can distalize a full cusp CL.II if the 8's are missing or extracted.
- BeneFit system: If you want to intrude the molars place the benefit arms gingivally (AOB cases), while more occlusally for extrusion (Deep bite cases).
- No need for bonding or braces for doing all these action with the BeneFit system.
- When we use a forsus, remove the cinch when we need distalizing, to allow the maxillary molars to distalize while bringing the lower arch forward to create additional spaces to alleviate crowding. If you have fixed appliance, you can leave the upper molars uncinched to let the molars distalize freely.

3. Extraction

- Extraction in class II is not necessary done when there is crowding only, if it can't be achieved by class II elastics, then extraction will always be an option to retract the upper teeth.
- Calculate how much overjet and crowding you have to decide how many teeth to extract (Upper only or upper and lower) (fig.35)

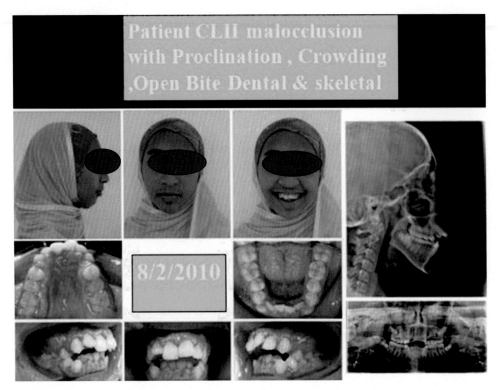

Fig.35 CLII adult with severe crowding, gingival hypertrophy, mouth breather

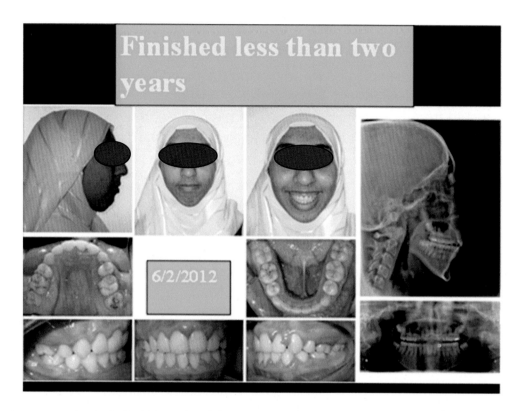

Finished less than two years

6/2/2012

CROWDING

SEVERE CROWDING

- If you have severe crowding and extraction is needed, you must calculate how much space you need.
  - ◦ 1) for retracting
  - ◦ 2) To relieve the crowding.

- When you retract 4mm you need double the space. Therefore, if you want to go from 6mm overjet to normal 2mm. (6-2) x2 = 8mm needed for retraction alone.

- The parameter can't be changed, if there is 8 mm deficiency of the arch you have to maintain that space. But the overjet can be manipulated.
  - Overjet can be manipulated by advancing the mandible which will help in correcting the OJ, you will need less space and less anchorage to retract. As the OJ will be corrected from both upper and lower. If the space with crowding and correction of over jet, we have to decrease the need for space by advancing the mandible and utilize the space by full anchorage.
  - **Whatever overjet you want to reduce, you need to multiply it by 2. To get the space required.**
  - Use the space to relieve the crowding first, then you can deal with the overjet.

- **Full cusp CL.II: full anchorage is a must + distalization in case you can't do mandibular advancement.**
- **TPA alone isn't enough anchorage.**

MILD & MODERATE CROWDING

- Start with a headgear, especially if the patient still in early adolescence, in order to distalize the molars and create space to help alleviate crowding.
- A Forsus can also be used after alignment. Excess wire can be left distal to the upper molars prior to placing a cinch to allow for a similar distalization effect as a headgear.
- When we align and bring the mandible forward but there is still a great amount of overjet, distalize the molar then starts to retract remaining teeth.
- If you're not in a heavy wire you must not use any force. There must be heavy wire in upper and lower, preferably SS. (elastics can be used)
- You gain some space by expanding using the arch wire during leveling and alignment.
- Crowding in the lower with increased overjet: proclining the lower can help.
- Extraction is preferable If proclination is excessive.

- Stop the habit (tongue crib)
- It's hard to place posterior bite plate in adult with open bite, as it's difficult for the patient to tolerate it.
- Either extrude upper (box elastics) or lower or intrude molars.
- If you want equal amounts of extrusion in both upper and lower then use a similar wire for both arches, whereas if you don't want any movement of the lower anterior teeth because of excessive gingival display etc. then use a heavier wire in the upper and a lighter wire in lower.
- If you don't want to extrude in the lower for any reason, reduced alveolar bone, gingival recession or mobility. Use a heavier wire in the lower and lighter in the upper.
- It's always preferred to extrude the upper anterior teeth and not the lower.
- If you want to extrude, but full closure of open bite will not be achieved, intrude posterior teeth.
  - By placement of TADs buccally with transpalatal bar 5mm away from the palate with a heavy wire.
  - Both 6+7 must be bonded and intruded.

- You can place TAD buccally and TPA palatally and pull from both sides so no tipping will occur on the molars.
- With TPA and TAD (fig.36)
  - If 7 is erupted, you have to include it in the intrusion system.

TPA with TADs Buccally

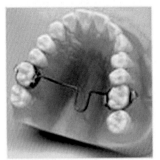

TAD's Buccally & Palatally

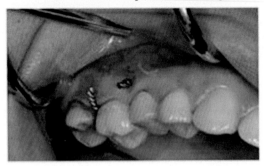

Fig.36

- After closing the anterior bite, evaluate whether you need extraction or not.
- Extraction in open bite will be favorable, as you will bring the posterior teeth more forward and the bite will close.
- CL.II + open bite: extraction (whether with or without crowding will be helpful)
- If the CLII, open bite is associated with any crowding, extraction is the best choice.

DEEPBITE

- Bringing the mandible forward will reduce the deep bite.
- Procline teeth, open the bite.
- Always treat vertical then AP. Reduce deep bite then treat it like a normal class II.
- Remember where the deep bite is coming from. Is it because of the upper teeth or lower teeth? (Increased curve of spee? or High lip line?)
- Any distalizing device opens the bite, because it extrudes the posterior teeth.
- In deep bite patients, try to avoid lower extraction unless it is necessary.
- Use anterior bite plate even in adults with fixed braces.
- Any retraction of the upper anterior teeth cannot occur if the deep bite is not treated.

CROSSBITE

- First thing is to determine whether it's skeletal or dental unilateral or bilateral.
- In the true posterior unilateral cross bite, check if the constriction is due the upper arch collapsing inward or lower arch outward, which determines the best way to correct it.
- Extraction can't be done before expansion! **<u>Never!</u> Always after**

POSTERIOR CROSSBITE

- Either hyrax or quad helix (bilateral) or by expanding the arch wire with inter maxillary cross elastics if it is not severe.
- Can be done dentally too, in young adults.
- In older adults, if you need more skeletal you can use MARPE. Therefore, done with TADs. Sometimes hyrax is appropriate even for adult especially if they do not have gingival recession.
- Hyrax: 2 bands, 2 on premolars and 2 on molars.
  - When you choose the bands, one side must be bigger than the other, so you can put the appliance in, as there is no path of insertion.
  - Therefore, when placed in, you have a little flexibility on the other side.
  - When expansion is done, alveolar bone will be expanded, and it will open the suture.

- *What do you see clinically when there is expansion?* Diastema.
- There will be more anterior expansion.
- Patients who have gingival recession: try to avoid tooth-borne expander as it will lead to buccal recession due to tipping. Thus, go for bone-borne expanders (TADs)
- For adults it is preferred to add TADs in the palate, either 2 or 4. To give a more skeletal effect.

- For MARPE, the force of expansion will go to the TADs that are inserted in the palate.
  - Less effect on the alveolar bone and more effect on the suture.
  - Therefore, side effects on teeth will be decreased e.g., recession.
  - MARPE can be done at any age, palate is fractured slightly and slowly to separate the suture.

- If you have good alveolar bone, no gum recession, good oral hygiene, and then you can do normal expansion with hyrax and no need for Marpe. (Very rare)
  - MARPE will decrease the chances of recession, therefore used in cases with thin biotypes.

- The problem in adults is how to maintain the expansion you have achieved.
  - Expansion must be maintained 6 months after treatment is done.
  - Heavy wire (Square arch form) must be placed and widened to prevent any relapse.

- Bilateral crossbite, with good balance, and because of a large mandible, the crossbite can be maintained. As relapse would occur and maxilla is of normal size.
- Types of expanders and effects:
  - Quadhelix – dentoalveolar, bilateral
  - Hyrax – skeletal and sutural opening
  - Arch wire- tipping for minor cases

- Archwire can be expanded, to maintain the results you got from expansion. Done using heavy wires.
- After expansion you must evaluate what you will do next. And what is needed to treat the Class II.
- Two things you must think about in class II, is how much you need to retract the canine and the anterior teeth and the OJ is increased. etc.

- For the early adult you can use forsus, but if it's not possible because of patient's age, then extraction must be done.
- Expansion will create more space too.
- Deep bite with expansion, is good as it will decrease the overbite. But with open bite, it's a problem.

CROWDING

- Mild crowding + CL.II + cross-bite: expansion then treat the CL II as explain above (AP)
- Severe crowding + CL.II + cross bite: expansion then extraction and start correction according to the severity canine position and OJ. We might need extra anchorage.
- CL.II + open bite + cross bite: expansion then extraction. This is favorable in correction of AP and to reduce the open bite (get rid of the cause of the open bite). We might need extra anchorage.

CROSSBITE AND DEEP BITE

- Favorable. A lot of the mechanics are favorable.
- Some devices that incorporate expansion and distalization simultaneously can be used in early adults.
- BeneFit system can be used for expansion and distalizing but mostly dentoalveolar because there is no jackscrew in the middle. Intrusion, extrusion, mesialization or distalization can be performed with this system.
- The more you distalize the more you will open the bite. "Scissor theory"
- Once you correct the deep bite, after reevaluation, you can determine whether you need extractions or not.
- Place your device on the 6, and it will push the 7 with it.

- After you reach to the right location for the 6 or 7, lock it with the Allen key, and then retract. If you remove it too early, the molars may relapse.
- If the cross bite is mild, can sometimes expand the arch wire and use crossbite elastics at the molar area from upper palatal to the lower buccal surfaces. This also causes extrusion of the posterior teeth, thus helping in correction of the deep bite as well.

CROSSBITE AND OPENBITE

- Stop the habit using a tongue crib.
- Expansion and then extrusion of the anterior teeth.
- Expansion same way as above but try not to use cross bite intermaxillary elastic during arch wire expansion.
- Check the open bite and the smile line. If gummy smile, do not extrude anteriorly but intrude posteriorly by TADs place buccally with tongue crib or transpalatal bar.
- If this is associated with crowding, extraction after expansion could be a choice for correction of the CLII and favorable for open bite closure.
- If the molars are full cusp CLII, maximum anchorage is needed (TADs)

In class II Division II

- Mostly associated with deep bite
- You must open the bite to get rid of the effect of the lip.
- With proclination you might not need any extraction.
- You must obtain optimal interincisal angle to prevent relapse.
- Get rid of the deep bite by extrusion of posterior teeth if possible.

3 principles you must know in CL II div.2:

Get rid of the cause (which is the effect of the lower lip)

Get a good Inter-incisal angle (by proclination of U & L incisors)

Get rid of deep bite by either extruding the molars or intruding the U incisors or/and L, depending on the lip line.

High risk of relapse if we do not follow the 3 principles.

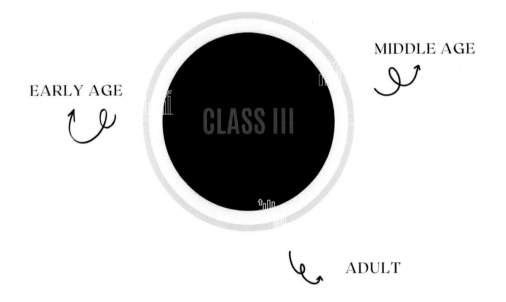

EARLY AGE

MIDDLE AGE

CLASS III

ADULT

Class III malocclusion is the least common type of malocclusion in many communities, accounting for approximately less than 5% of all cases.

Highest incidence of class III malocclusion is observed among Japanese and Koreans. In class III malocclusion the mesiobuccal cusp of permanent maxillary first molar occludes interdentally between the mandibular first and second permanent molars, instead of occluding with mesiobuccal developmental groove of the permanent first molar.

In this type of malocclusion, the mandibular incisors overlap the maxillary incisors instead of the other way around.

This reverses the normal anteroposterior relationship of the incisors and sometimes called as "reverse overjet".

In class III malocclusion, maxillary and mandibular canines do not exhibit any contact with each other.

ETIOLOGICAL FACTORS

- Heredity
- Unilateral/bilateral hyperplasia of mandibular condyle
- Occlusal premature contact
- Enlarged adenoids.
- Habitual forward positioning of the mandible predisposes to pseudo-class III malocclusion.
- Premature loss of deciduous molars.

DIAGNOSIS

Diagnosis of class III malocclusion should be aimed at evaluating whether the condition is dental or skeletal and true or pseudo-class III malocclusion.

The diagnosis should be based on clinical examination and radiographic evaluation of skeletal growth pattern using lateral cephalogram.

TREATMENT

The main treatment objectives in Angle's class III malocclusion may include:

- Reduction of crowding
- Correction of the reverse overjet
- Correction of incisor overbite
- Correction of molar relationship.

1. TREATMENT OF PSEUDO-CLASS III MALOCCLUSION

Pseudo-class III malocclusion can be treated by eliminating occlusal premature contact and other local factors.

Various types of orthodontic appliances used to treat class III malocclusions in pre-adolescent.

2. TREATMENT OF ANTERIOR CROSSBITE

Anterior crossbite in class III malocclusion can be treated by using lower anterior inclined planes or removable orthodontic appliance incorporating expansion screw designed for anterior expansion.

3. TREATMENT OF POSTERIOR CROSSBITE

Posterior crossbite in class III malocclusion can be treated by rapid maxillary expansion.

CHAPTER VII / CLASS III- EARLY AGE

- The treatment will take a very long time.

- Continuous treatment required until growth is completed.

- If patient comes at this early age, it can be either hereditary or early closure of cranial suture.

- It can also be due to a habit (mouth-breathing), if so, then stop the habit

- Early closure of cranial suture from any condition e.g., syndromes, leading to a small maxilla and large mandible.

- In syndromes like Crouzon's, these surgeries must be done early as it will affect the growth of the brain too. These syndromes should be well managed as early as possible.

- Hereditary: can start with pseudo class III with shift due to a premature contact, or no shift and true class III.

- Class III patients will always grow in a class III tendency.

- First device to be used at this age is the chin cup. As anterior teeth and 6's might not be fully erupted.

- Chin cup will hold the mandible while it allows the maxilla to grow. It will redirect the growth of the mandible. At this time, when you're holding the mandible back, the tongue might go up and push the maxilla & premaxilla which can stimulate anterior growth.

- Chin cup can't be used for more than 2 years. Why? Because it has an extraoral part that is placed on the head that might affect the growth of the skull as well. Loss of hair, and skin irritation might also be seen with prolonged use of a chin cup.
- With chin cup, reevaluation will be needed in every stage.

Appliances with different age groups: Our Plan is.

- Chin cup – early (fig.37a, b)
- Bionator – mixed dentition (early and middle) (at the transitory period from deciduous to permanent dentition) (Fig.38)
- Reverse headgear/facemask preferable in mixed or late mixed dentition (but can also be used in any earlier stage) (with expansion if needed)
- Upper and lower fixed appliances and elastics (permanent dentition)
- Surgery (always inform parents to keep the door open for surgery, especially the hereditary type)

Pseudo Class III is usually due to a premature contact so for treatment we start with chin cup and URA with recurve spring to procline the anterior teeth.

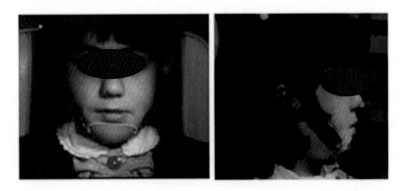

Fig.37a.b Chin cup is used in the first stage of treatment of CJ III

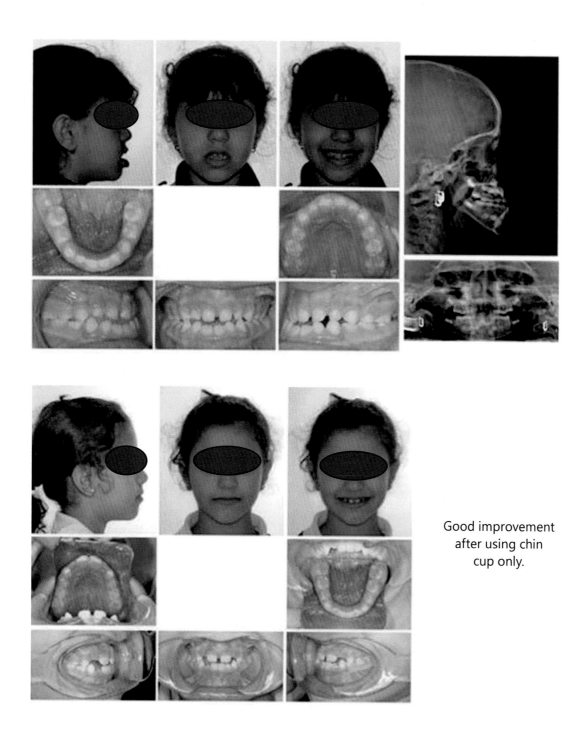

Good improvement
after using chin
cup only.

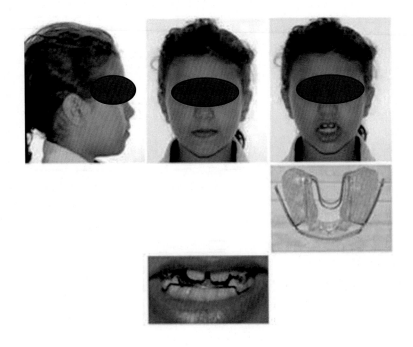

Fig.38 Using Bionator CL III in early age after the eruption of the upper central.

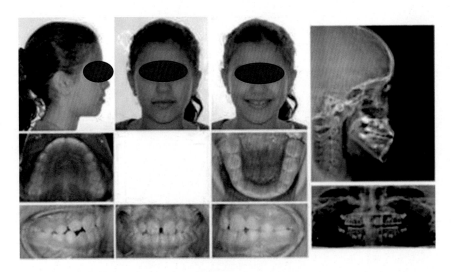

After using the Bionator CL III

CROWDING

- With mild crowding or severe crowding, evaluation is needed.
- Any kind of choice of treatment whether extraction or not, will affect the treatment of the class III in the future.
- Never do early extraction in early age to solve the crowding and then assess the class III.

MILD/MODERATE CROWDING

- relieve by expansion & proclination.

SEVERE CROWDING

- Procline and expand then wait till you correct the class III.

OPENBITE

- Worst situation with class III
- If you use chin cup it will increase the vertical height and cause more opening of the bite.
- Habit must be checked and stopped. Especially with mouth breathing and low position of the tongue which might lead to an enlarged mandible.
- If the habit is pushing the maxilla forward, leave it.
- Habit breaker can be used, to prevent the tongue from moving forward. Which can also be used with a vertical pull chin cup if possible
- With the habit breaker, we can start the 2x4 utility arch with internal helices to procline and extrude the upper incisors.

DEEPBITE

- Favorable, as the devices used will open the bite.
- In deep bite with erupted incisors, you use a chin cup and removable appliance.
- Hawley with recurve spring to procline incisors.
- Chin cup will increase vertical height, and removable appliance will procline which will also open the bite.
- When you jump the occlusion, you can use the same device for retention.
- Double check the over lapping of the incisors after jumping the anterior cross bite

CROSSBITE

- Most class III are associated with a crossbite as the maxilla is small.
- Anterior crossbite is a given as its class III.
- In many cases it is associated with posterior crossbite too. Due to the small size of the maxilla.
- Before you do expansion check the patient's cast because it may not need expansion laterally.
- The expansion with a hyrax can be done in 2 weeks (1 or 2 turn per day, each turn 0.25mm)
- Sometimes when you see a patient in an early mixed dentition, and anterior teeth are present and 6's are present, face mask can be used, to pull the maxilla forward.
- Hooks can be present in the bonded hyrax to be used for the facemask, which is mesial to the canine and distal to the lateral, (between canine and lateral) to pull from near center

of resistance of the maxilla. The bonded hyrax design with PBP is helpful in jumping the occlusion.

- Bite plane will open the occlusion. Advantage of bonded hyrax would be to open the bite too while pulling the maxilla.

  ◦ This also depends on the compliance of the patient for the following devices.

- When to use chin cup and reverse HG (facemask)
- Never leave the patient without a device.
- Bionator class III, can be used for pseudo class III. (fig.39)
- Bionator class III, can be used to maintain the results achieved by the first stage. To hold the upper and lower together.
- **Hold the upper and lower together at every stage.**
- The acrylic will hold the teeth together and the tongue will be directed to the maxilla and may help stimulate further growth.
- Bionator class III, can be used sometimes as the first phase, which will help push the anterior segment forward and hold the mandible in its place.
- Myofunctional appliances will keep the upper and lower together but won't direct the tongue to the premaxilla like the Bionator III.
- Most dangerous period of class III, is the prepubertal and pubertal stages.

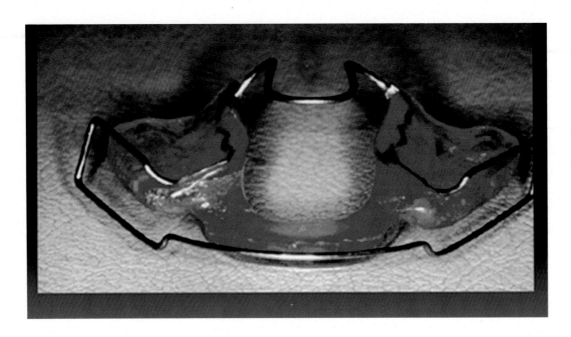

Fig.39 Bionator CLIII

CHAPTER VIII / CLASS III - MIDDLE AGE

IT is a very critical period for the CLIII, we start to fight against the growth so if we did not see the patient before this period and we did not solve the problem then this is the best stage for using a reverse HG/Face mask to bring the maxilla forward and to hold the mandible from further growth. This is a very important period because it is before the peak of growth. We can manage some pseudo CLIII's with 2x4 and expansion screw, with Utility arch without face mask (fig.40).

In order to carry the maxilla forward with the face mask, the best intra oral device is the hyrax with bands on the 6`s & 4`s with extended arms palatally to the centrals, even if it is bonded hyrax. It is necessary to have extended arms palatally behind upper centrals because when we pull the maxilla it has to be pulled in one block, if there are no extension arms, the whole buccal arch will shift mesially and might create crowding.

Quadhelix with extended arms to the centrals might help sometimes especially if some cases in which we need a 2x4 to move the anterior teeth while we are protracting the maxilla.

CROWDING

- Leave treatment for crowding for later when the maxilla and mandible will be in an acceptable position.

Stage of treatment for this age

- Reverse HG to pull as much as possible and mandible must be held in position as much as possible in this period as there is more growth. Need patient compliance to bring maxilla forward then we take care of a crowding according to where the maxilla will be in relation to the mandible. We will treat the crowding accordingly as mild, moderate & severe as before. The classification will be based on the results of face mask use (fig.41)

OPENBITE

- Unfavorable, because any protracting to the maxilla face mask will increase the open bite by clockwise rotation of the maxilla and mandible.
- Bonded hyrax can be used to decrease the open bite by intrusion of the posterior teeth with the help of the posterior bite plane.
- Stop the habit which might be the main cause of the open bite
- Same sequence done like early age.
- Hyrax will also help with breaking the habit.
- Mouth breathing should be referred to ENT.

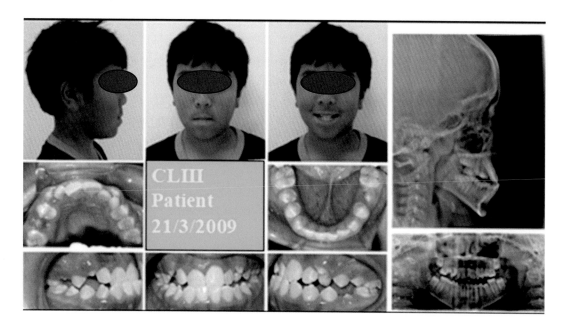

Fig. 40 CL III patient with mild crowding upper only need bi lateral expansion using Hyrax and antero-posterior expansion using Utility arch.

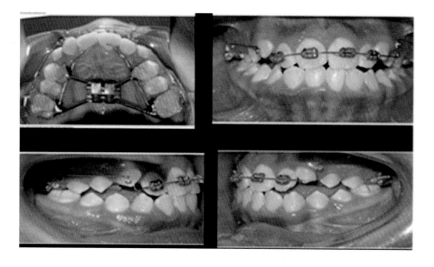

CLIII crowding Rx expansion by Hyrax, AP by 2x4 Utility arch.

CLIII crowding Rx expansion by Hyrax, AP by 2x4 Utility arch.

Always leave the door open for surgery. As growth can be unpredictable and relapse might occur.

- If the OB doesn't close automatically, go for a utility arch to extrude the anterior teeth and close the bite if you have bands on 6`s. This cannot be done with a bonded hyrax. In that case, finish the traction of the maxilla then deal with closing the open bite (AP first then vertical)
- Most common problem with class III is open bite because after protraction of the maxilla we have to create a good over jet and overbite to prevent relapse.

DEEPBITE

- Favorable because the protraction of the maxilla will open the bite and reduce the deep bite and it will have a good overbite after successful maxillary traction with the face mask.

CROSSBITE

- Check if there is crossbite when you advance the maxilla on your study models.
- Always check your study model if you have cross bite after that.
- If there is no crossbite expansion won't be required, otherwise we will get a scissor bite.
- Sometimes expansion is done with protracting the maxilla if needed to correct the cross bite, it will facilitate bringing the maxilla forward. (Mobilize the maxilla sutures)
- Some techniques, opening for 2 weeks and closing for 2 weeks can be done to help facilitate the above point. (This happens when patient doesn't have crossbite).
- When you are protracting the maxilla at this age, and eruption of permanent teeth is still present. If 4s are not present, bonded hyrax can be used. If there are bands on the 4, a hook is placed on the bands of both 4 & 6.
- If no hooks are available, place kobayashi hooks, but elastic placed on the bracket not the kobayashi, it will just prevent the extra oral elastic from slipping.

- It is preferable as you can use 4 sites to protract the maxilla. (You will pull on the whole maxilla)
- Hyrax must be maintained for retention.
  - Positioner must be used to maintain the results and the relationship between maxilla and mandible.

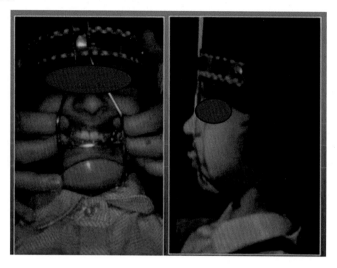

Fig.41 Reversed Head gear (face mask) used with intra oral device (Hyrax)
to pull the upper arch forward and hold the mandible

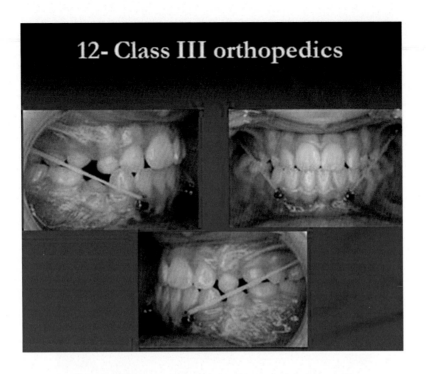

Fig.42 Skeletal Plates with CL III for elastics camouflage
to bring maxilla forward mandible back in a young adult

Most important thing with class III is to bring the maxilla as fast as possible forward, Especially in this PRE-PUBERTAL PERIOD.

CROSSBITE WITH MODERATE CROWDING

- Expansion with proclination will both create space, in cases of class III with retroclined incisors. Correct the AP first then deal with crowding.
- Even in severe crowding do not hasten for extraction. AP first

CHAPTER IX / CLASS III – ADULT

1) ORTHODONTIC TREATMENT

- In the 14-16 age group, the reverse HG with the hyrax expand plate can still be used, as there is still a little growth to protract the maxilla.

- After growth at 18-20 or above, camouflage can be done, with fixed appliance upper and lower. (fig.43a, b)

  - o   Depends on the severity, if the ANB is –2 you can camouflage with fixed appliance and extract only in the lower.

  - o   Face mask can be used in any of these ages but requires high compliance of the patient. It will give only dentoalveolar effects in adults.

  - o   The new technique is by using skeletal plates on the lateral side of the chin and skeletal TADs in maxilla in the Zygomatic area.

  - o   If soft tissue is already camouflaging the CLIII feature, we still can also camouflage the dental arches as well.

  - o   Try always to keep the upper dental arch intact without extraction because teeth hold the full size of the dental arch and that what we need in CLIII.

- If surgery can't be done, then extraction with fixed can be an option: lower or upper & lower.

- Upper & lower fixed appliances with skeletal TADs for the mandible to retract the whole mandibular arch and inter maxillary elastics to bring the maxilla forward.

- In surgical cases, try to avoid extraction as much as possible. (OR DON'T) Esp. when surgery is decided, do not extract in lower arch. Decompensation might be done by extraction in the upper then correct by surgery
- Prepubertal and Pubertal is the most dangerous part for class III.
- With fixed upper and lower, class III elastics can be done to maintain results.
- If the patient comes to the clinic at this age, most of the growth has already been done. Growth can occur in the mandible up to 17-18 years of age in males.
- Maxilla can be protracted 10mm by surgery (maximum), but we should always remember that if only the maxilla should be brought as that much then it will affect the nose size looks flatter. It is preferable for bi-maxillary surgery when correcting such a discrepancy. Lefort 1 maxillary advancement and BSSO for lower is usually performed. Never perform a mandibular setback alone. 100% relapse will happen and will reduce the space for the tongue and airway.

CROWDING

MILD & MODERATE CROWDING

- Expansion in upper arch can be done if needed, with a face mask.
- Procline upper teeth to create space and camouflage class III, with fixed appliance and class III elastics.
- A good amount of overjet and overbite must be obtained to prevent relapse of class III.
- Extraction can be done in the lower but not the upper arch, as it will be needed for camouflage.
- Extraction in lower is favorable but not upper.
- When decompensation is done prior to surgery, retroclination will be done of the upper anterior teeth, and reverse OJ will be created.
- If surgery is decided from the beginning. Avoid extraction except in the upper only to decompensate for surgery.

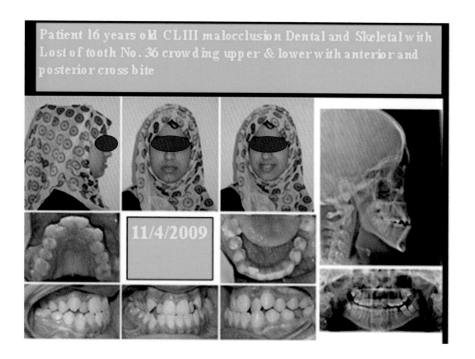

Fig.43a CL III skeletal & dental treated by face mask to pull the maxilla forward, hyrax intra orally

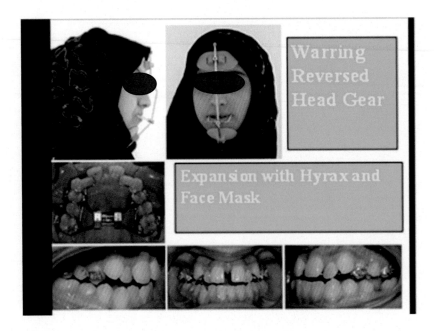

Fig.43b Hyrax show the need for expansion of the palate in creating spacing between centrals which we need during traction of the maxilla

SEVERE CROWDING

- If extraction is done in the upper, extraction in the lower must be done too. This is only done in cases of camouflage. (fig.44a, b)

- Extraction of upper 5 and lower 4. Unless enough anchorage is not available, depends on every case.

- Correct the crowding by extraction together with correction of the AP relation with the help of inter maxillary CLIII elastics.

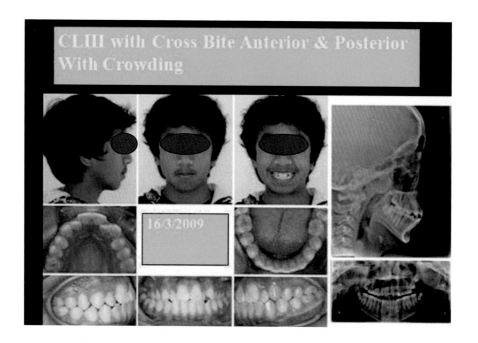

Fig.44a

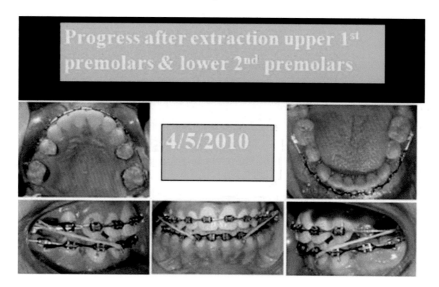

Fig.44b CLIII crowding with extractions U&L premolars upper 5s lower 4s

- First stop the habit by tongue crib etc. if it does exist, mouth breathing or tongue thrusting (fig.45a, b)

- Create an overjet first. (AP first then vertical)

- If there is a gummy smile, extrusion of upper incisors shouldn't be done. Extrusion of lower incisors or intrusion of molars. Always after correction of AP

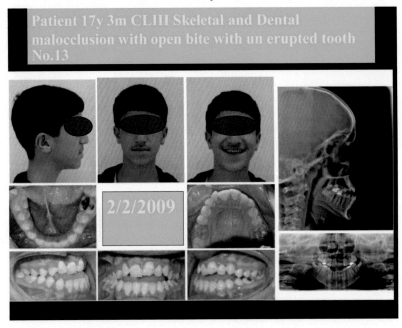

Fig.45a CL III malocclusion with open bite skeletal & dental, mouth breathing, crowding.

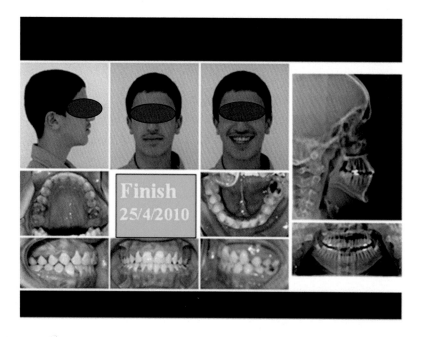

Fig.45b CLIII open bite Rx with face mask & fix appliance inter maxillary elastics

- If the hyrax is present, cut the arms and leave the screw. TADs can be added to it and connect it to 6 and 7. And that will lead to intrusion of the molars closing the bite.

- Every open bite must have enough overjet prior to closing the open bite.

- If surgical, open bite should not be closed. It will be corrected by surgery.
    - Surgery is done in 3 pieces. It is not done in one piece.

- 3 segment surgery in Le fort 1. Correction Ap. And vertical maybe associated with BSSO.
    - Anterior segment can be lowered (tipped downwards), while the posterior segments can be impacted.
    - This is preferred over closing the open bite with orthodontics alone.
    - 3 segments are more stable and can be manipulated more.

- Protraction with face mask with hyrax can be done, and overjet created, it is favorable. (fig46a, b)

- As the deep bite can be used to camouflage. Proclination can be done by placing posterior bite raisers to jump the bite, and then remove it.

  ◦ It will compensate the amount of deep bite used while proclining.

  ◦ Overbite is the best thing for retention of class III.

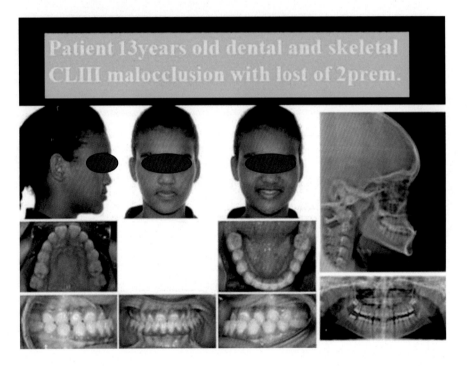

Fig.46a

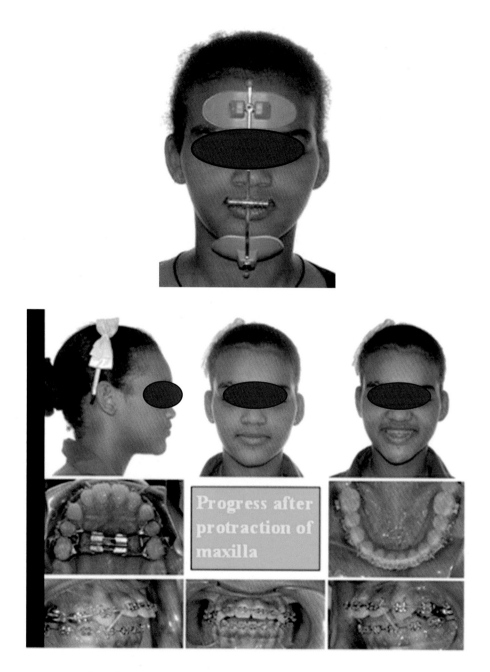

Fig.46b CL III skeletal & dental using face mask and hyrax

DEEPBITE WITH CROSSBITE

- Favorable as you can expand and that will reduce deep bite expansion with the protraction of the maxilla will facilitate the maxilla movement forward.

DEEPBITE WITH CROWDING

- Try to minimize extraction.
- **Mild & moderate:** expansion + proclination will help and improve the condition.
- **Severe:** extraction after correction of AP

CROSSBITE

- If its bilateral in adult leave it (without shift) check on study model if patient still can use face mask with hyrax after AP correction again, we can reevaluate the need more for expansion.
- In case of camouflage the expansion can always be done by MARPE or SARPE.

2) ORTHODONTIC- SURGIRIES FOR CLASS III

- It is always better to do bi-maxillary surgery as it is more stable
- If one jaw it will be only in the upper but never only in lower jaw
- Most of surgical orthodontic cases is preferable to have surgery first then ortho. Treatment
- Females – 18 years.
- Males – 21 years.

surgical case with orthodontic by expansion with hyrax, fix U&L appliances and only one jaw surgery by maxillary advancement (fig.47a, b, c)

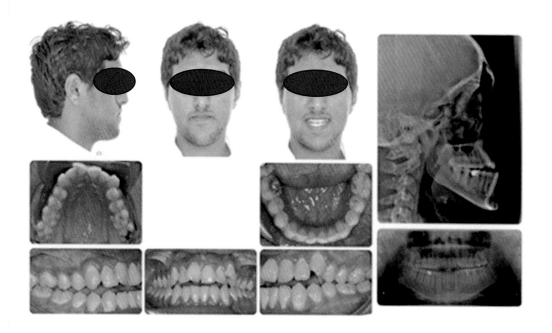

Fig.47a CL III treated by expansion with RME hyrax with fix appliance U&L

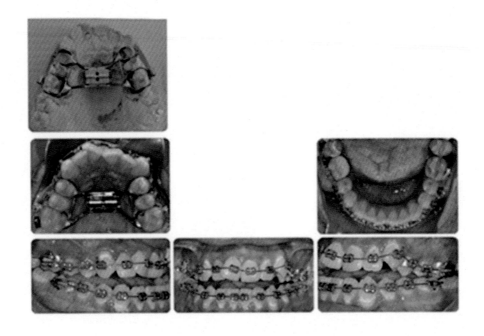

Fig.47b RME hyrax expansion of the maxilla with fix U&L

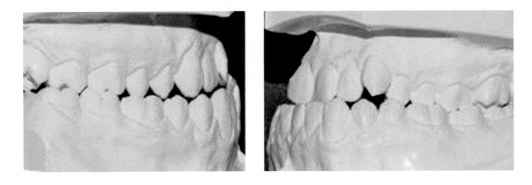

Negative over jet

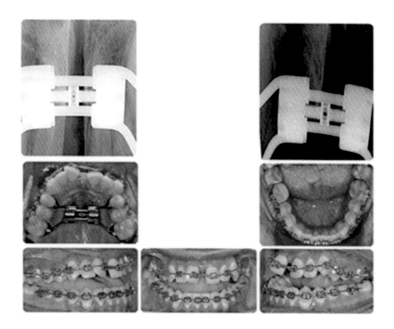

Expansion was sufficient for relieving crowding and for palatal surgery to close the cleft.

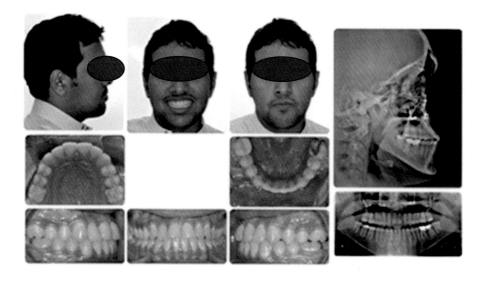

Fig.47c CL III one jaw surgery only maxillary advancement

CLIII with cleft lip and palate.(fig.48a,b,c,d)

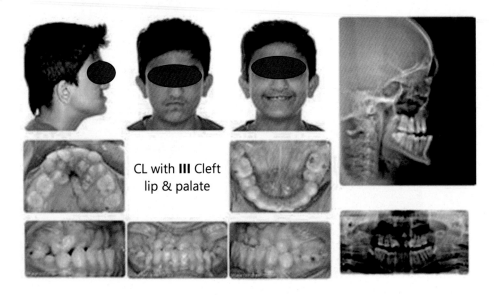

CL with **III** Cleft lip & palate

Fig.48a Patient with CL III with cleft lip and palate. None of the recommended surgeries had been performed.

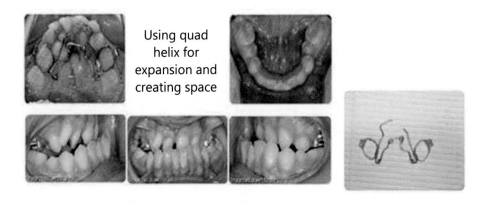

Using quad helix for expansion and creating space

Fig.48b we start to expand the area for a bone graft using a quad helix for expansion.

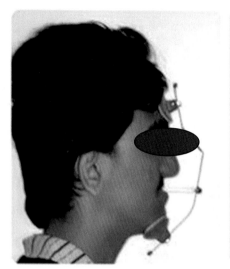
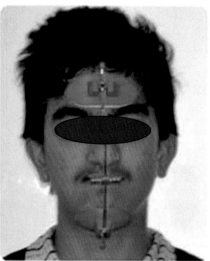

Fig.48c using a facemask with fixed upper & lower appliance
with extraction of lower 4s to camouflage the CL III

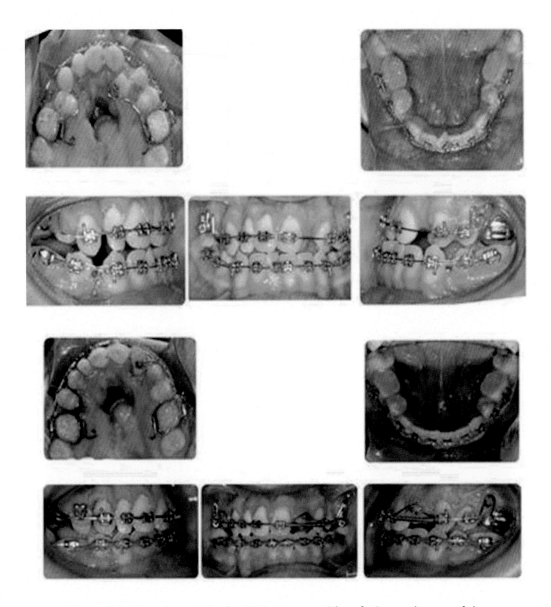

Fig. 48d Patient done only the ABG surgery with soft tissue closure of the palate and refused orthognathic surgery for the skeletal CL III.

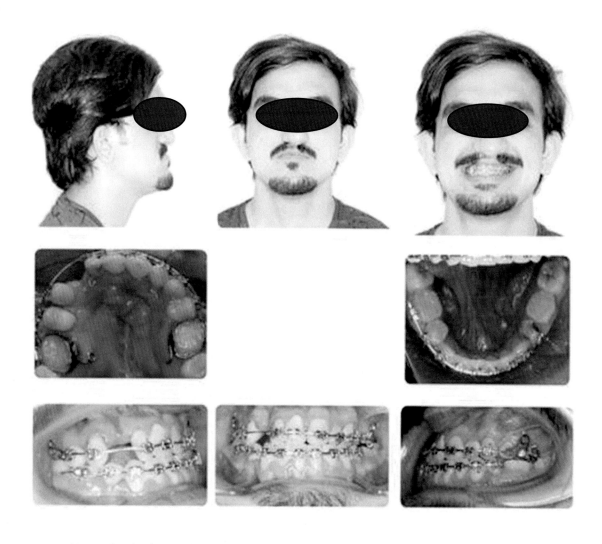

Expansion by hyrax showing a clear suture opening in the middle of the palate

CHAPTER X / ANCHORAGE

DENTAL ANCHORAGE

1) Tip the molars distally using a tip up bend in the arch mesial to molar tube. +

2) Torque the molar root in a cortical bone. +

3) Add more teeth- increase no. to your anchored teeth ++

WIRE BENDING ANCHORAGE

1) Torque for anchorage teeth and tipping for moving teeth. +

2) Make a stop sharp (omega shape) in front of the molar tube. ++

3) Tip up at end of the arch wire to tip molar distally against movement. +

DEVICES

1) Head gears (cervical, high pull, combination, Face mask) will require compliance. +++

2) All types of bite plane if required. ++

3) TPA or/and any modification (tong crib, Nance). ++

4) All expanders if needed in the case (Quadhelix, hyrax on 4 teeth+++, W). ++

5) All types of inter maxillary elastics. ++

6) TADs (palate, buccal, skeletal). +++

According to effectiveness: High+++, Medium ++, Low +.

CHAPTER XI / RETENTION

REMOVABLE APPLIANCES

APPLIANCE	CASES
Hawley	Expansion cases Deep bite cases Existing of little spacing (for build up or not)
Reversed Hawley	Same in above but mainly with canine buccally
Wrap around	All above and mainly after spacing closure. For better settling
Essix (clear tray)	used for all type of treatment. Must cover all teeth (including 8's if erupted)
Fix retainer	used mainly in the lower from canine to canine. Or/and premolar to premolar in extraction case Later to lateral in the upper in closing diastema

CHAPTER XII / SUMMARY

AGE	PROBLEM		TREATMENT
			Class I
Early age	Crowding	Mild	1) **Removable with expansion screw.**
			2) **Slicing of C mesially (if needed)**
			3) **Proclination with Hawley+ recurve spring or 2x4 appliance + Utility arch w/TPA**
		Moderate	**Expansion + proclination (a must here)**
			1) **Removable with expansion screw.**
			2) **Slicing of C mesially (with retention for molars)**
			3) **Proclination with Hawley+ recurve spring or 2x4 appliance + Utility arch w/TPA**
		Severe	**Serial extraction (CD4E)**
	Anterior Openbite	Mild Crowding	**Extrusion will give space.**
			1) **Stop the habit and correction occurs on its own.**
			2) **If not, 2x4 appliance + utility arch + extrusion bend +TPA**
			3) **Ismail's Appliance**

Age	Problem		Treatment
		Moderate Crowding	1) Stop habit then re-evaluate.
			2) Slicing or expansion
		Severe crowding	1) Stop the habit.
			2) Serial extraction (TPA to prevent mesialization of 6)
	Posterior Openbite	Mild Crowding	1) Frankel or Myobrace
	Deepbite	No crowding	1) ABP with URA
		Mild & Moderate Crowding	1) ABP with URA
			2) Expansion, proclination, slicing.
		Severe crowding	1) ABP (treat deepbite)
			2) Extraction + TPA sometimes 2x4 to intrude incisors
	Crossbite	Single tooth	1) Removable with Z-spring + Adams clasp + I clasp (<2mm)
			2) Fixed 2x4
		Group	1) Removable with recurved spring or with segmented screw.
			2) Fixed
	Anterior Crossbite	Mild crowding	1) Solve crossbite (proclination, removable or 2x4)
			2) Expansion for more space
		Moderate crowding	1) Fix crossbite same as previous (posterior bite plate if >2mm)
			2) Follow by slicing
		Severe crowding	1) Fix crossbite.
			2) Extract C then procline.
			3) Serial extraction if very severe

Age	Problem		Treatment
		Deepbite	1) **Posterior bite plate and procline with removable or 2x4 plus bite raiser.** 2) **Remove PBP and place ABP. to solve deep bite**
	Posterior Crossbite		True Unilateral (no shift): **Expansion on affected side only with removable + Screw or Quadhelix.** False Unilateral (with shift): **Expansion bilaterally with removable + screw (posterior bite plate if needed) or bonded hyrax.** Bilateral: **Expansion bilaterally with removable and screw or bonded hyrax**
		Mild crowding	1) **Treat crossbite with expansion, which will give space as well.**
		Moderate crowding	1) **Hawley + Recurve spring maybe slicing**
		Severe crowding	1) **Expand then evaluate if serial extraction is needed.**
		Deepbite	1) **Expansion (dental – quadhelix, skeletal – bonded hyrax)** 2) **Then treat deepite. Expansion will help here.**
		Openbite	1) **Stop habit.** 2) **Expansion (PBP if needed) by quadhelix, W-arch or bonded hyrax.** 3) **Reduce the open bite**
		Openbite+ mild/mod Crowding	**Crowding will be solved when expansion or extrusion is done. (Space will be gained)**
		Openbite+ severe Crowding	**Extraction might be needed (favorable) after solving open bite**

Age	Problem		Treatment
Middle age	Crowding	Mild	1) **Expansion (same as previous)** 2) **Proclination with recurve spring or 2x4 appliance** 3) **Slicing of E's**
		Moderate	1) **Expansion + Proclination with recurve spring or 2x4 appliance + Slicing of E's**
		Severe	1) **Serial extraction** 2) **Check the canine position**
		Anterior open bite	1) **Stop the habit.** 2) **Mild + moderate: 2x4 appliance w/ utility arch (for proclination + extrusion)** 3) **Severe: serial extraction with above.**
		Posterior openbite	1) **Frankel or Myobrace** 2) **Then treat crowding normally**
		Anterior crossbite	1) **2x4 appliance + posterior bite raiser**
	Deepbite		1) **ABP and determine cause.** 2) **2x4 appliance + utility arch + intrusion bend (upper problem)** 3) **2x4 appliance + with anterior bite plan**
		Mild/mod crowding	**ABP fix.** **Mild: proclination with intrusion** **Mod: proclination + slicing of C `s**
		Severe	1) **Open the bite with ABP then continue Rx normally** 2) **Extraction**

AGE	PROBLEM		TREATMENT
	Anterior Crossbite	Crowding	**>2mm: open bite with PBP or bite raisers it depends either URA or fix.** **Mild: procline** **Mod: procline and slice C`s** **Severe: Extraction**
	Posterior crossbite		**True Unilateral (no shift): Expansion on affected side only with removable +expansion Screw or Quadhelix.** **False Unilateral (with shift): Expansion bilaterally with removable + screw (posterior bite plate if needed) or bonded hyrax.** **Bilateral: Expansion bilaterally with removable and screw or bonded hyrax**
		Deepbite	**ABP fix with expansion widening of the arms for expansion.**
		Openbite + Severe crowding	1) **Get rid of the habit.** 2) **Expand according to previous rules.** 3) **Extraction at the end, if needed.**
Adult	Crowding	Mild	1) **IPR last thing to be done.** 2) **proclination with wire if profile allows**
		Moderate	1) **Widening arch with wire** 2) **Extraction if needed.** 3) **IPR last thing to be done.**
		Severe	1) **Extraction (4 premolars) Fix appl. U&L**

Age	Problem		Treatment
	Anterior Openbite		1) Stop habit if any. 2) Determine problem from which arch and where to extrude/intrude. 3) Fix w/ extrusion bends or box elastics
		Severe crowding	1) Treat cause 2) Extraction 3) TADs to intrude, TAD+TPA, TPA but away from palate
	Deepbite	Crowding	First treat deepbite then crowding. 1) ABP with intermaxillary elastics to extrude molars. 2) Anti-curve of spee in the lower
	Anterior Crossbite	Crowding	1) Fixed upper +lower. 2) >2mm posterior bite raisers or PBP 3) Mild & Mod: Proclination will give space. 4) Severe: procline + align, crossbite then deal with crowding extraction if needed.
	Posterior Crossbite	Crowding	First treat crossbite then treat crowding like above. True Unilateral (no shift): In mild cases quadhelix or wire + cross elastics False Unilateral (with shift): Hyrax or quadhelix Bilateral: Hyrax or MARPE

Age	Problem		Treatment
		Anterior Openbite	**Treat crossbite -> AP -> Vertical** 1) **Bonded hyrax (intrude posterior and expands)** 2) **Surgery in severe cases.** 3) **Hyrax with bands and or TPA expand then buccal TAD`s to intrude posterior teeth to get rid of the deep bite.**
		Deepbite	**Crossbite first as mentioned above, then deepbite.** **Banded hyrax will help open bite. Never bonded hyrax.**
			Class II
Early age	No crowding		**Expansion 1-2mm to cause autorotation of mandible with URA**
	Crowding	Mild	1) **removable appliance with expansion screw (1-2mm)**
		Moderate	1) **Removable with expansion screw, or recurve spring.** 2) **Slicing of Cs and Ds** 3) **Headgear if maxillary incisors are severely proclined.**
		Severe	1) **Expansion to get class I by autorotation.** 2) **Headgear, then reevaluate for serial extraction.** 3) **Serial extraction**

Age	Problem		Treatment
		Crossbite	**True Unilateral (no shift): Expansion on affected side only with removable + Screw or Quadhelix.**
			False Unilateral (with shift): Expansion bilaterally with removable + screw (posterior bite plate if needed) or bonded hyrax.
			Bilateral: Expansion bilaterally with removable and screw or bonded hyrax
			Expansion here is more than above.
		Crossbite +severe crowding	**Expansion, then evaluate for serial extraction.**
	Openbite		1) **Stop habit, closure on its own.** 2) **2x4 appliance and tongue crib (no compliance)** 3) **When openbite closed, deal with it like a normal class II.** 4) **Posterior bite plate used if expansion is done.**
		Mild crowding	1) **Expansion for autorotation of mandible** 2) **Posterior bite plate for intrusion of posterior teeth**
		Moderate crowding	1) **Expansion** 2) **More space needed: slicing**
		Severe Crowding	1) **Expansion** 2) **Check canine position.** 3) **More space needed: slicing or extraction Cs** 4) **Above is not enough: serial extraction.**

Age	Problem		Treatment
	Deepbite		**Div. 1: ABP (inclined) with expansion** **Div. 2: ABP (inclined) with expansion + recurve spring for proclination**
		Anterior crossbite	1) **PBP + recurve spring + expansion screw** 2) **The ABP + Treat deep bite**
		Posterior crossbite	True Unilateral (no shift): **Expansion on affected side only with removable + Screw or Quadhelix.** False Unilateral (with shift): **Expansion bilaterally with removable + screw (posterior bite plate if needed) or bonded hyrax.** Bilateral: **Expansion bilaterally with removable and screw or bonded hyrax** **Crossbite -> crowding -> reevaluate if distalization is needed.**
Middle age			*Critical time for treatment of class II*
			1) **Change Div. 2 to Div. 1 by recurve spring and expansion for 6 months.** 2) **If there no time for expansion, then use twinblock and expand with it.** 3) **Problem from Max: use headgear.** 4) **Problem from Mand: Functional appliance** 5) **We always prefer do advance mandible than distalize maxilla in CLII** 6) **Remember always this age is the best for using FA as pre peak of growth**
	Crowding		1) **Solve class II then crowding. By FA to reduce OJ**

Age	Problem		Treatment
		Mild & Moderate	**Mand retruded: little expansion, Functional appliance, if needed 2x4 appliance** **Max protruded: Headgear, 2x4 appliance**
		Severe	1) **Treat AP** 2) **Extraction** 3) **Check canine position**
		Severe OJ+ crowding	1) **Reduce OJ with functional appliance.** 2) **Then crowding. Extraction if needed**
	Openbite	Mild & moderate	1) **Tongue crib + 2x4 appliance., utility arch** 2) **Functional appliance (FRANKLE) or high pull headgear**
		Severe	1) **Habit breaker to treat open bite.** 2) **Extraction if needed and 2x4 appliance**
	Deepbite		**-Functional appliance:** 1) **Open the bite (trim posteriorly if needed), occlusally or oblique.** 2) **Procline lower anteriors by FA reduce deep bite.** **-Cervical Headgear.**
		Mild & moderate	1) **Treat class II** 2) **Treat Deepbite (FA or HG)** 3) **Then treat normally the crowding**
		Severe	1) **Treat class II** 2) **Treat Deepbite (FA or HG)** 3) **Extraction of upper 4's or U&L**

Age	Problem		Treatment
		Div. 2	1) Inclined ABP (serves as FA)
			2) Procline anterior teeth Recurve spring URA & ABP
			3) 2x4 appliance with utility arch inclined fix ABP
	Crossbite		1) Severe skeletal: Expansion with Hyrax (no time to waste here)
			2) Dental: Quadhelix can be used
			3) Mild and Maxilla is at fault: expand with inner bow of HG.
			4) Then functional appliance with expansion for mand. advancement
			5) Tapered maxilla: Quadhelix
		Mild & Moderate	1) Expansion like mentioned above.
			2) Treat AP then crowding
		Severe	1) Expand first and keep hyrax for retention.
			2) Functional appliance If still before the peak
			3) Re-evaluate if extraction is needed. If yes, extract 4s.
		Openbite	1) Expansion (will act as habit breaker).
			2) Extrusion of anterior or bonded hyrax to prevent opening the bite further and intrude posterior teeth.
			3) Then HG or FA (FRANKLE) as needed.
		Deepbite	1) Expansion with hyrax (banded can be used if 4 is erupted)
			2) If above is not enough, inclined ABP. (acts as FA) and maintain expanded arch

Age	Problem		Treatment
Adult	1) 1) **Mandibular advancement: - Fixed functional appliance (full cusp class II) Forsus or Herbst - Class II elastics (1/2 cups class II)**		
	2) 2) **Distalization: Carrier, Headgear, Beneslider, Benefit, distaljet**		
	3) 3) **Extraction**		
	Crowding	severe	1) **Extraction**
			2) **Relieve crowding then deal with overjet**
		Mild & moderate	1) **Distalize molar (will create space)**
			2) **Slight expansion with archwire**
			3) **Proclining lower incisors (if crowding is there)**
	Openbite		1) **Stop habit.**
			2) **Extrude upper or lower incisors (both elastics/heavy wire) or both or intrude molars (TPA, TPA+TADs, TADs).**
			3) **Extraction (whether with or without crowding)**
	Deepbite		1) **Procline teeth**
			2) **Distalize (forsus/distal jet) will open bite.**
			3) **Determine reason for deepbite and treat accordingly.**
	Crossbite		1) **First treat the crossbite**
			Young adults: hyrax (skeletal + dental) or quadhelix (dental effect)
			Older adults: MARPE (with tads)
			Minor crossbite: Heavy archwire
			2) **Forsus in younger adults or extraction if not possible**

Age	Problem		Treatment
	Crowding		**Mild: expansion then AP forsus elastic CLII** **Moderate AP and might need stripping.** **Severe: expansion then evaluate for extraction**
	Deepbite		1) **Expansion** 2) **Distalize (benefit)** 3) **Last evaluate if extraction is needed.** 4) **Full cusp CLII in general heed full anchorage TAD`s**
	Openbite		1) **Stop habit.** 2) **Expand** 3) **Extrude Ant. or intrude post. according to case**

Class III

- **Chincup: early mixed dentition.**
- **Bionator: early and middle mixed dentition.**
- **Reverse HG (Facemask): Late mixed dentition.**
- **Upper and lower fixed appliance & class III elastics: permanent dentition.**
- **Surgery: too severe. Always an option.**

Age	Problem		Treatment
Early Age	Pseudo class III		1) **Chincup and removable appliance with recurve spring.** 2) **Bionator class III**
	Crowding	Mild & moderate	1) **Expansion with removable appliance.**

Age	Problem		Treatment
		severe	1) Procline and expand with removable appliance.
			2) Wait till correction of class III is done before any extraction.
	Openbite		1) Stop habit or habit breaker (bite will close)
			2) Chin cup vertical pull can worsen the openbite??
	Deepbite		1) Chin cup
			2) Hawley with recurve spring
			3) Retention: same devices
	Crossbite		1) Bonded Hyrax with facemask if 1, 2, 6 are present.
			2) Bionator III
			3) Myobrace (retention)
Middle age	Crowding		1) Treatment of class III with facemask (reverse HG)
			2) Crowding is dealt with after class III Rx.
	Openbite		1) Stop habit.
			2) Bonded hyrax with face mask (expansion slightly and intrusion of molars)
			3) 2x4 with utility arch (if doesn't close on its own)
			4) AP first then vertical
	Deepbite		1) Reverse HG with hyrax extended arms.
			2) 2x4 appliance upper
			3) With utility arch
	Crossbite		1) Bonded Hyrax with facemask.
			2) If banded is used, hooks on 4's and 6's.
		Crowding	1) Expansion will create space. Face mask to correct AP

Age	Problem		Treatment
Adult			14-16 years: reverse HG and TADs/plates 18-above: camouflage or surgery
	Crowding	Mild & moderate	1) **Expansion if needed.** 2) **Fixed with class III elastics.** 3) **Extraction in lower but not upper**
		Severe	1) **Extraction (if done in upper must be done in lower)**
	Openbite		1) **Stop habit correct AP.** 2) **Intrude molar or extrude incisors by fixed.** 3) **Surgery if not possible.**
	Deepbite		1) **Proclination with fixed + posterior bite raisers.**
		Crossbite	1) **Expansion (procline and reduce bite)**
		Crowding	Mild: **expansion and proclination** Severe: might need extraction **with AP correction**
	Crossbite		Young adults: **hyrax (skeletal + dental) or quadhelix (dental effect)** Older adults: **MARPE (with tads)** Minor crossbite: **Heavy archwire** **ANY OF THE ABOVE MALOCCLUSION IF IT WAS DECIDED FOR SURGERY SHOULD HAVE DIFFERENT TX PLAN** Decompensation exo. on upper only and not lower prefer surgery BIMAX, upper Max. only never LOWER only

REFERENCES

- Proffit WR: Contemporary Orthodontics, 4th edition, Mosby-Elsevier, 2007

- Graber TM, Vanarsdall RL: Orthodontics Current Principles &Techniques. Mosby, 2000

- Nanda R: Biomechanics in Clinical Orthodontics WB Saunders Co, 1996.

- Gianelly A, Goldman HM: Biologic basis of orthodontics. Lea & Febiger, 1971

- Clark WJ: Twin Block Functional Therapy. Mosby 2002

- Systemized Orthodontic Treatment mechanics MBT September 2007

- Barrer HG: Orthodontics: The State of the Art. University of Pennsylvania Press. 1981

- Salzmann JA: Orthodontic in daily practice

- Jarabak & Fizzell: Light wire Edge wise Appliances

- Tweed Charles H: Clinical orthodontics

- Cheol -Ho Paik In-Kwon Park Tae-Woo Kim, Orthodontic Miniscrew Implants ScienceDirect 2009

- RM Ricketts 1976 Bioprogressive therapy as an answer to orthodontic needs part II -NCBI

- Aldo Carano, Stefano Velo, Cristina Incorvati, Paola Poggio Clinical applications of the Mini-Screw-Anchorage-System (M.A.S.) in the maxillary alveolar bone, PROGRESS in ORTHODONTICS 2004; 5(2): 212-230

- Orthodontic retainers and removable appliances: principles of design and uses By (author) Friedy Luther, By (author) Zararna Nelson-Moon .Dec.2012

- Orthodontic functional appliances. Theory and practice; Padhraig S. Fleming (author), Robert Lee (author) Hardback (24 Jun 2016)

Printed in the United States
by Baker & Taylor Publisher Services